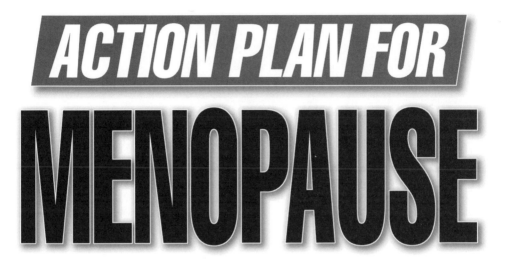

ACTION PLAN FOR MENOPAUSE

BARBARA BUSHMAN, PhD
JANICE CLARK YOUNG, EdD

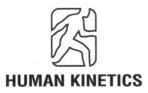

HUMAN KINETICS

Library of Congress Cataloging-in-Publication Data

Bushman, Barbara Ann.
  Action plan for menopause / Barbara Bushman, Janice Clark Young.
    p. cm.
  Includes bibliographical references and index.
  ISBN 0-7360-5618-1 (soft cover)
  1. Middle aged women--Health and hygiene. 2. Physical fitness for middle aged women.
  3. Exercise for middle aged women. 4. Menopause. I. Young, Janice Clark. II. Title.
  RA778.B965 2005
  613.7'045--dc22

                           2004027991

ISBN: 0-7360-5618-1

Acquisitions Editor: Martin Barnard; **Developmental Editor:** Leigh Keylock; **Assistant Editor:** Kim Thoren; **Copyeditor:** Patricia L. MacDonald; **Proofreader:** Kathy Bennett; **Indexer:** Betty Frizzéll; **Permission Manager:** Carly Breeding; **Graphic Designer:** Fred Starbird; **Graphic Artist:** Francine Hamerski; **Photo Manager:** Dan Wendt; **Cover Designer:** Jack W. Davis; **Photographer:** Barbara Bushman, unless otherwise noted; **Art Manager and Illustrator:** Kareema McLendon; **Printer:** United Graphics

ACSM Publication Committee Chair: Jeffrey L. Roitman, EdD, FACSM; **ACSM Communications and Public Information Committee Chair:** Harold W. Kohl, PhD, FACSM; **ACSM Group Publisher:** D. Mark Robertson; **ACSM Editorial Manager:** Lori A. Tish

Human Kinetics books are available at special discounts for bulk purchase. Special editions or book excerpts can also be created to specification. For details, contact the Special Sales Manager at Human Kinetics.

Printed in the United States of America   10 9 8 7 6 5 4 3 2 1

Human Kinetics
Web site: www.HumanKinetics.com

United States: Human Kinetics
P.O. Box 5076
Champaign, IL 61825-5076
800-747-4457
e-mail: humank@hkusa.com

Canada: Human Kinetics
475 Devonshire Road Unit 100
Windsor, ON N8Y 2L5
800-465-7301 (in Canada only)
e-mail: orders@hkcanada.com

Europe: Human Kinetics
107 Bradford Road
Stanningley
Leeds LS28 6AT, United Kingdom
+44 (0) 113 255 5665
e-mail: hk@hkeurope.com

Australia: Human Kinetics
57A Price Avenue
Lower Mitcham, South Australia 5062
08 8277 1555
e-mail: liaw@hkaustralia.com

New Zealand: Human Kinetics
Division of Sports Distributors NZ Ltd.
P.O. Box 300 226 Albany
North Shore City
Auckland
0064 9 448 1207
e-mail: blairc@hknewz.com

I dedicate this book to my dad, Kenneth, and the memory of my mother, Josephine (1934-2003), who taught me to dream high, work hard, and find joy in each day.

Barbara Bushman

I dedicate this book to my parents, Martha and Dale Robinson, for the values and work ethic they taught me.

Janice Clark Young

CONTENTS

ACKNOWLEDGMENTS

Thanks to our spouses, Tobin Bushman and Frank Young, for their continual understanding, support, and patience during the research leading to and the writing of this book.

Thanks to Sarah Scheerer for assistance with compiling background material, Joan Newman for reviewing our rough drafts and giving insightful comments, and Brenda Goodwin for being such a great model (and role model) for us.

We appreciate the cooperation of the Springfield Greene County Park Board for allowing us to use their workout rooms and equipment for the photographs found in this book.

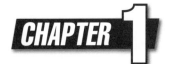

CHAPTER 1

THRIVING WITH HORMONAL CHANGES

Menopause. Does that word elicit worrisome thoughts? Considering some of the terminology used in the past—"the change"—it does sound a bit ominous, but it is a natural part of aging. Do you worry about how your body will change? As a woman, you progress through many phases during your reproductive life, and menopause is an entirely expected, normal process. Do you wonder what is happening in your body to produce symptoms of hot flashes or vaginal changes? Do you have questions on how to find ways to not just survive but to also thrive during these changes? The answers to these and other questions are covered in this chapter and the following chapters as you develop an action plan for menopause.

The word *menopause* was first used by physicians in 1821 (Ballard 2003). The Greek origins are *menos*, which means month, and *pausos*, which means ending. Menopause is, therefore, the cessation of the monthly menstrual cycle. On average, menopause occurs at 51.3 years of age for women in the United States, but the range is between 40 and 55 years of age (Wilson 2003). It is interesting to note that the onset of menopause has remained around the age of 50, as recorded since the time of ancient Greece.

Considering that in the United States more than 40 million women are postmenopausal and another million plus will join them each year, you are not alone in facing these changes. With the baby boomer generation (born between 1946 and 1964) turning 50, the rate of those entering menopause is increasing. You will experience this time in your own unique way, and we hope you will consider how this transition can be a time to flourish and an opportunity to improve your health and fitness.

Stages of Menopause

Menopause is part of the natural progression of your reproductive life, starting years ago with menarche (the first menstrual cycle), which typically occurs around the age of 12 or 13. The time of puberty until menopause is termed by some as the premenopause phase. During this time, menstruation (also known as your period) occurs approximately every 28 days. Perimenopause (also known as climacteric or menopausal transition) begins before menopause and is a time of physical and hormonal changes. Menopause is the point of your last period, although by definition you have not experienced "menopause" until it has been one year following your last menstrual cycle. Perimenopause includes the time leading up to the last menstrual period as well as the following year (Goldman and Hatch 2000). Postmenopause refers to the time period following menopause (and thus is verified 12 months after the last menstrual cycle). The sequence and overlap of these time points are illustrated in figure 1.1.

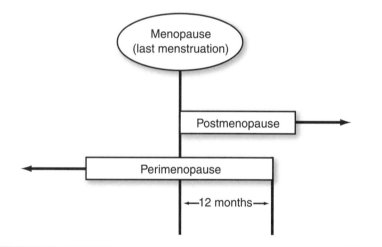

Figure 1.1 Menopause time line.

Historically, menopause has been viewed negatively. This is not surprising considering that in the early 1900s the life expectancy was not much different from the time of menopause. Thus, many women did not experience menopause or much of postmenopausal life before death. Currently, with the life expectancy for women at more than 80 years, menopause is no longer associated with the end of a woman's life. Actually, many women will spend approximately one-third of their lives postmenopause (Best Clinical Practices 2002). The main purpose of this book is to lead you to an active and healthy life during perimenopause and continuing into postmenopause. The word *menopause* may include the concept of "ending," but it is merely the end of the reproductive phase. We hope you will see a bright future in the time leading up to and following menopause.

Physiological Changes

During a woman's life, her body undergoes many changes. Reproductive hormones govern changes starting with menarche, through puberty, and into her adult life. These functional changes are brought about by hormonal alterations that will result in the physical changes and consequences discussed in this section.

Hormonal Changes

Estrogen is produced by the ovaries in various forms (estriol, estrone, and estradiol). Estrogen is the hormone responsible for changes in female sexual characteristics at puberty and is also related to other functions in the body, including bone health. The ovaries also produce progesterone. Regulation of the menstrual cycle occurs due to progesterone along with hormones released from a structure in the brain called the pituitary gland. Progestin is another term often used and is synonymous with progesterone.

The pituitary is activated to release follicle-stimulating hormone (FSH) and luteinizing hormone (LH) in a cyclic fashion by a control center of the brain, the hypothalamus. These two hormones move in the bloodstream from the pituitary gland to their target organs, the ovaries. FSH functions as its name suggests—stimulating follicular growth, or, in other words, signaling the growth of a group of cells that surround a developing egg (out of approximately 500,000 potential immature eggs). An increase in LH in the blood then provides hormonal information to the ovaries to release that egg (i.e., ovulation occurs). This monthly pattern of development of a follicle and the release of an egg happens over and over throughout a woman's reproductive life.

Estrogen is released from the follicular cells in the ovaries and in turn acts on the uterus to prepare for a potentially fertilized egg. This hormone also exerts feedback on the hypothalamus to decrease the stimulation of the pituitary gland, causing FSH and LH levels to decrease. After the egg is released at ovulation, the remaining follicular cells (now termed the corpus luteum) continue to produce estrogen and also, to a greater extent, progesterone. Progesterone continues the work of estrogen in the uterus to prepare for a fertilized egg (increased blood supply; glandular support; and cell growth of the inner lining of the uterus, called the endometrium). In the absence of a fertilized egg, the levels of progesterone and estrogen decline as the corpus luteum naturally breaks down. This results in the breakdown of the lining of the uterus and the beginning of menstruation.

The rise and fall of all these hormones (FSH, LH, estrogen, and progesterone) provide for menses each month, unless pregnancy occurs or other health-related concerns interrupt this orchestration. The hypothalamus acts as a conductor, signaling the pituitary gland and the ovaries in a rhythmic fashion that repeats each month. During perimenopause, the precise monthly rhythm of hormones becomes less regular. Hormone levels begin to change as the ovaries decrease in size. As menopause approaches, the follicles in the ovaries are no longer able to respond to the stimulus from FSH and LH, so estrogen (most specifically estradiol) levels drop and progesterone release is basically zero. The main type of estrogen remaining after menopause is estrone, which is a weaker form of estrogen. Estrone is produced within fat tissue and will increase with age and with the amount of fat in the body. Thus, just as at puberty, hormone changes bring about continued physical changes for the female body during menopause.

Physical Consequences of Hormonal Changes

Because of changes in the monthly rhythm of hormones just described, a number of physical changes occur during menopause. It has been suggested that characteristics associated with menopause should relate to these hormonal changes rather than just include symptoms associated with aging in general (Goldman and Hatch 2000). Treatment options for the various physical changes should be considered in light of each woman's risk profile, which includes family history as well as current health status, in consultation with a physician aware of the complete picture.

Alterations in Menstrual Bleeding

Changes in menstrual bleeding may occur during perimenopause (Goldman and Hatch 2000). Menstrual cycles can become irregular, and your periods may include heavy bleeding. It is thought that these changes may be due to lower levels of estrogen that may be insufficient to stimulate the LH spike to trigger ovulation (i.e., an anovulatory cycle—menstrual bleeding occurs, but no egg was actually released). The estrogen that is still available causes the uterine lining to grow, but without progesterone, this continues for a longer time than normal. This may result in a heavy period when the woman's period does occur as a result of the eventual dip in estrogen. Heavy menstrual bleeding may also be caused by a sustained (but slower) increase in estrogen. Ovulation still occurs, but the time in which estrogen exerts its influence on the uterus is longer (thus increasing the inner lining), so the menstrual period that follows is heavy and more prolonged.

Variability in the time between menstrual periods tends to increase during perimenopause (National Institutes of Health [NIH] 2002). Ovulation may become intermittent, and cycle length can vary from fewer than

21 days to more than 35 days. Menstrual bleeding can occur at regular intervals but can be very low in volume or can be excessive. Some women experience frequent and excessive bleeding without any cyclic pattern.

Changes in your menstrual cycle may be due to these perimenopausal changes, but ruling out other causes is reason to consult with your physician. Abnormal uterine bleeding could also be a sign of cancer of the reproductive tract or some other systemic disorder, such as blood-clotting disorders, liver disease, or kidney failure (NIH 2002).

Hot Flashes

A hot flash has been defined as "the increase and perception of heat within or on the body" (Goldman and Hatch 2000, 1158). This feeling of heat can be in the upper part of your body (face, neck, and upper torso) or body-wide. Hot flashes are often accompanied by perspiration and sometimes red blotching of the skin. When this occurs during sleep, it is termed a *night sweat*. The term *vasomotor symptoms* is used within the scientific community as a global term to include both hot flashes and night sweats (North American Menopause Society [NAMS] 2004).

Hot flashes appear to be one of the first signs of perimenopause and may continue for two years into postmenopause (possibly longer for some women). The frequency appears to be very individual but typically occurs in a pattern for a given woman—it might be weekly or even hourly (NAMS 2004). Approximately 75 percent of women will experience hot flashes (NAMS 2004). Hot flashes can be brief (1 minute or less) or long (12-plus minutes), although most last 1 to 5 minutes (about 7 percent are longer, and about 17 percent are shorter) (NAMS 2004).

Various factors seem to be associated with hot flashes, including the following situations (NAMS 2004):

- Warm environmental temperature
- Cigarette smoking (one more good reason to quit or not to start)
- Low physical activity

Anecdotal reports of certain foods (especially hot foods—either hot in temperature or spiciness) or beverages (such as alcohol or those with caffeine) triggering hot flashes have not been supported with research studies at this point.

The physiological cause of hot flashes is not known and actually may involve multiple factors rather than just one. Estrogen levels may be a factor, as well as other hormones associated with nervous system function. The control of core body temperature is another likely contributor. Some research would suggest that around the time of menopause, women develop an increased sensitivity to heat caused by a narrowing of the thermoneutral zone (Freedman and Krell 1999). In other words, a smaller temperature change will cause the body to try to cool itself by dilating blood vessels in the skin, resulting in flushing and perspiration. Thus, hormonal levels, changes in nervous system, and alterations in temperature maintenance in the body may all be involved in causing hot flashes (NAMS 2004).

What can be done to cope with hot flashes? Lifestyle modifications have been recommended by the North American Menopause Society (NAMS). One such recommendation is to find ways to keep body temperature in the normal range. If small changes in core temperature can trigger a hot flash, then it follows that keeping core temperature low would be beneficial. Lowering air temperature, using a fan, eating or drinking cool foods and beverages, and dressing in layers (so you can adjust your individual temperature) may be helpful. Some lightweight sleepwear products have been developed that wick moisture away from the body to keep you drier when night sweats are a problem.

Women who exercise regularly have reported fewer and less severe hot flashes than did sedentary women (Hammar, Berg, and Lindgren 1990). In addition, those with higher physical activity levels had fewer hot flashes than did less physically active women in another study (Gold et al. 2000), so the amount of activity may be important. In women who had reported at least five hot flashes a day, exercise did bring on a hot flash when they attained a certain sweating level. However, other postmenopausal women who had no symptoms (i.e., reported never having a hot flash) remained free of hot flashes during exercise that elicited sweating (Freedman and Krell 1999). It appears that "although strenuous activity may elicit hot flashes in unconditioned women, daily exercise is associated with an overall decreased incidence" (NAMS 2004, 13). Thus, observational studies suggest a benefit for women committed to a regular exercise program. Additional research is needed to determine the optimal exercise program for reducing the incidence and severity of hot flashes.

Relaxation techniques may be beneficial in reducing hot flashes. Paced respiration (slow, deep breathing from the abdomen) appears to potentially reduce the frequency of hot flashes (Freedman and Woodward 1992). Women in these studies were taught slow, deep breathing and implemented that technique when they felt the onset of a hot flash. Fifty percent fewer hot flashes were noted when this technique was used (Freedman et al. 1995).

Nonprescription remedies abound, although many have not been shown in clinical research studies to be beneficial compared with a placebo treatment (a placebo is an inactive substance that results in a perceived reduction in symptoms) (NAMS 2004). Soy compounds have been studied because they contain isoflavones (compounds that may have estrogen-like effects). Comparisons and recommendations regarding the use of soy products are difficult because of the variety of products available to consumers as well as the differences in actual amounts of isoflavones available within products. Most studies used 40 to 80 milligrams of isoflavones per day and have shown only a slight reduction in hot flashes. It is currently not known whether supplementing with isoflavones is safe in women with breast cancer. Black cohosh (commercial preparation Remifemin) has shown benefits in some studies but produced no improvements in other studies. Long-term effects are not known, as studies have been relatively short in duration (less than six months), although the incidence of side effects appears low when taken for less than six months (NAMS 2004). Evening primrose oil has not been studied extensively, but current research does not support its effectiveness in decreasing the number of hot flashes. Reported side effects of evening primrose oil include nausea and diarrhea (NAMS 2004). Topical progesterone creams have various formulations, and research studies have not consistently shown benefits for hot flashes, although some positive effects have been noted.

Some women with persistent hot flashes may need prescription medications. Estrogen and estrogen plus progestin have both been shown to effectively relieve hot flashes in many research studies (NAMS 2004). Women with an intact uterus should take a progestogen (which is a natural or synthetic hormone substance that produces effects similar to those of progesterone) along with estrogen to prevent problems with the inner lining of the uterus (excessive growth of the cells in the endometrial, or inner, lining of the uterus and potentially endometrial cancer). Hormone therapy is contraindicated in women with any of the following: a history of hormone-sensitive cancer, liver disease, history of blood-clotting disorders, and confirmed cardiovascular disease (NAMS 2004, 21). The potential side effects of hormone therapy include uterine bleeding, breast tenderness, nausea, abdominal bloating, fluid retention in the extremities, headache, dizziness, and hair loss (NAMS 2004, 21). Progestogen alone may be helpful for treatment of hot flashes, although the safety with regard to breast cancer risk is not yet known.

Low-dose oral contraceptives (combined estrogen and progestin) are commonly prescribed for women desiring both contraception and relief from hot flashes. As with all medications, there are contraindications (i.e., reasons a person should not use the medication), including history of blood clots, cardiovascular disease, migraine, hormone-sensitive carcinoma, jaundice, or liver disease as well as smoking for those over the age of 35 (NAMS 2004, 22). For more information on hormone therapy, see the sidebar on page 8.

Nonhormonal prescription therapies are also being investigated for their influence on hot flashes, even though the government approval is for another health concern. Drugs in this category include certain antidepressants (e.g., venlafaxine and paroxetine [Stearns et al. 2003]), the anticonvulsant gabapentin, and older antihypertensive drugs (clonidine and methyldopa). Each medication has side effects and contraindications for use. Research in this area continues. You should discuss your options, in light of your symptoms and health history, with your physician.

Sorting Out the Research on Hormone Therapy

The Women's Health Initiative (WHI) study has resulted in much media attention on the disadvantages of hormone therapy. The WHI is very comprehensive and includes multiple "arms," or substudies. Two separate arms were stopped: One using a combination estrogen and progestin (trade name Prempro) was stopped prematurely in 2002 (16,608 postmenopausal women participated), and the other using only estrogen (trade name Premarin) in a group of women who had hysterectomies was stopped prematurely in 2004.

In the estrogen plus progestin study (E+P), women taking the hormones had more heart attacks, strokes, blood clots, and breast cancers at 5.2 years into the study compared with those taking a placebo (Writing Group for the Woman's Health Initiative 2002; Wassertheil-Smoller et al. 2003; Chlebowski et al. 2003). Thus, it was concluded that E+P does not give a woman cardiovascular protection but may actually increase the risk of heart attack or death caused by coronary heart disease (Manson et al. 2003). The combined E+P therapy was initiated after menopause (note that some of the women had been on hormone therapy in previous years, and the mean age was 63.2 years of age). Some suggest the timing of initiation of hormone therapy may explain the increased heart disease noted in this study; previous observational studies had suggested a protective effect or at least a neutral influence. The influence of a high body mass index (BMI was 28.5 in these women, which is classified as overweight) also deserves consideration. Benefits were fewer incidences of colorectal cancer (Chlebowski et al. 2004) and fewer hip fractures (Cauley et al. 2003).

Other studies not associated with the WHI also found an increased risk of breast cancer with the use of E+P, regardless of whether the progestin was taken continuously or discontinuously (some women take the progestin only a certain number of days per month) (Li et al. 2003). The use of E+P appears to also increase breast density, which in turn makes accurate mammography more difficult (Gann and Morrow 2003). Changes in breast density may be a factor to consider (Gann and Morrow 2003).

In the estrogen-only (E) arm of the WHI study, there was again an increased risk of stroke, but on the positive side, a decreased risk of bone fracture (Women's Health Initiative Steering Committee 2004). The E therapy was neutral in its effect on heart disease (the risk was neither increased nor decreased) (Women's Health Initiative Steering Committee 2004). The women in the E study had already undergone hysterectomies, and researchers do not know at this time if health factors may differ for those without a hysterectomy.

Further analysis of these studies, including future follow-ups with the women involved, will help researchers and doctors, and individual women, determine the best course of action. These studies used two specific drugs, so it is still unknown if lower dosages of the drugs, other formulations, or even different methods of administration would be more (or less) beneficial (Writing Group

2002). In addition, research in the area of genetic studies of "estrogen receptor variants" is helping scientists understand the complex relationship between estrogen and heart disease (Hopkins and Brinton 2003, 2319).

Interpreting the current research may seem confusing and even frustrating at times. Different kinds of studies give different types of information. Observational studies involve simply observing a group of people over time to see what diseases may develop. For example, some of the research on physical activity and hot flashes examined differences in hot flash frequency in sedentary women versus active women. This helps provide insight, but some underlying differences between the two groups (other than just activity level) could also potentially explain differences in hot flashes.

A randomized controlled clinical trial (such as the WHI) involves many volunteers assigned to either a treatment group or a control group. In the WHI study, the treatment group was taking hormone therapy, while the control group received a placebo. Such research is reported in terms of absolute or relative risk. Relative risk compares the likelihood that a woman on hormone therapy will have a particular disease with the likelihood that a woman in the control group will have the disease. If the chance is the same in both groups, then the relative risk is 1.0, or an equal risk. In the WHI study looking at E+P, the relative risk for these women was 1.29, or a 29 percent increased risk of heart attack. Relative risk does not tell the whole story, however. Absolute risk looks at the actual number of disease cases that resulted from (or were prevented by) the treatment. The absolute risk of heart attack in the WHI study was 7 more cases in 10,000 women for those taking E+P. Having both the relative *and* the absolute risk is helpful for seeing the whole picture.

At this time, indications for hormone therapy include treatment of hot flashes, vaginal atrophy (local estrogen products formulated for use in the vagina could potentially be considered rather than pills), and postmenopausal osteoporosis (although nonestrogen medications should be considered—see the sidebar on page 16 for more information on these other medications). Estrogens and progestins do not appear to be appropriate for prevention of heart disease.

So, what if you are considering hormone therapy to help deal with menopausal symptoms? The American College of Obstetricians and Gynecologists (ACOG) recommends hormone therapy for the shortest time possible and in the smallest dose for the relief of symptoms; regular visits with your physician to review your status; and regular breast exams and periodic mammograms (ACOG 2002). Although a universal answer would probably be appreciated, it is impossible to give a simple answer to the question of what is right for you. The need to consult your physician in light of your individual health situation and family history is vital. The research in this area is moving forward, and new developments will be forthcoming. Staying in contact with your physician is a positive step in a healthy direction, whatever your decision regarding hormone therapy.

Vaginal Changes

As estrogen levels decrease, the lining of the vaginal wall becomes thinner and less elastic. In addition, vaginal secretions diminish, and pH of the vagina changes from what was typically acidic to alkaline. This shift in pH makes a woman more prone to vaginal infections.

Water-soluble vaginal moisturizers can be a helpful treatment for vaginal changes. Note that moisturizers are intended to act on the tissue of the vaginal wall to make it less dry, while vaginal lubricants (e.g., K-Y Jelly) are intended to provide lubrication during intercourse. When vaginal changes are severe, estrogen therapy may be recommended as a means to restore the thickness and elasticity of the vaginal walls. The FDA has approved estrogen in any form for this use (pills, patches, creams, or a vaginal ring).

Sleep, Memory, and Mood Changes

Other changes occur around the time of menopause. You may experience menopause-related sleep problems. Disturbances in sleeping are likely related to night sweats. You may be awakened by night sweats and be unable to return to sleep. Even if you do not awaken, your sleep may be disturbed (Joffe, Soares, and Cohen 2003). A regular exercise program is recommended for reducing stress and improving sleep quality (NAMS 2003).

Also consider your sleep routine. Small changes you make in your approach to sleep may reward you with a restful night. Try to avoid the following:

- Heavy meals late at night
- Alcohol, caffeine, and nicotine
- Exercise too close to bedtime
- Other activities in the bedroom, such as watching TV

Other suggestions to improve sleep include creating a relaxing environment that is quiet, cool, and dark. Keep a regular sleep schedule as much as possible, including getting up at the same time (even on weekends). For those with continued sleep disturbances, consultation with your physician is appropriate to rule out other disorders (e.g., allergies, thyroid problems, anemia, breathing problems such as apnea) (NAMS 2003).

With age, you may also experience memory problems—especially short-term memory. Whether these changes are associated with changing hormone levels or are simply due to general effects of aging is not fully known. Both men and women do experience short-term memory problems during middle age.

Other potential changes in your mood or behavior are also unlikely to be linked physiologically to menopause. "There are no scientific studies that support the belief that natural menopause contributes to true clinical depression, anxiety, severe memory lapses, or erratic behavior" (NAMS 2003, 12). Shifts in mood may be related to many factors, including sleep disturbances (and the associated fatigue) or other stresses in life that go hand in hand with the approach of menopause. For example, changes may occur in the family unit, such as children moving away or aging parents becoming more reliant on you. You may juggle many roles within your family in addition to work responsibilities and community involvement. The issue of stress and how to deal with it is covered in detail in chapter 7.

Positive Effects of an Exercise Program

Although your body changes in many ways during menopause, the benefits of an exercise program include those universally available to men and women as well as specific benefits related to menopause. For example, positive effects on physical fitness as well as improved quality of life (including areas related to physical mobility, pain, sleep, energy, social isolation, and emotional reactions) were noted in a recent study of postmenopausal women who were involved in six weeks of endurance exercise (bicycling), posture exercises, strengthening exercises (using elastic bands and free weights), balance exercises, and stretching (Teoman, Ozcan, and Acar 2004). Exercise can also be helpful in dealing with some symptoms of menopause, as discussed earlier in this chapter. The research evidence for decreased incidence of or at least less severe hot flashes was encouraging. Benefits related to cardiovascular disease as well as osteoporosis, depression, and cancer are also of direct importance to women.

Decreases Risk of Cardiovascular Disease

Cardiovascular disease (CVD) kills more women than any other disease. In the United States, "more than 500,000 women die of cardiovascular disease each year, exceeding the number of deaths in men and the next seven causes of death in women combined" (Franklin and Chinnaiyan 2004, 50). After menopause, the incidence of CVD increases steeply for women (NIH 2002). Before menopause, estrogen helps reduce the risk of heart disease in women. During and after menopause, the risk of heart attacks increases among women to a level that is equal to or greater than that of men.

Risk factors refer to "characteristics found in healthy individuals that have been observed in epidemiological studies [research studies of large groups of people] to be related to subsequent occurrence of CVD" (NIH 2002, 142). Risk factors for heart disease include age, family history, abnormal cholesterol and triglycerides, cigarette smoking, hypertension (high blood pressure), diabetes mellitus, obesity, lifestyle (including diet, physical activity, psychosocial factors, alcohol), high homocysteine (an amino acid found in the body that is thought to damage the lining of arteries and alter blood clotting), and elevated C-reactive protein (a marker of inflammation) (NIH 2002). This is quite a complex list. For our purposes in this book, we will focus on physical activity. Note that it is listed under "lifestyle," which is very appropriate—we want you to make regular activity part of your life.

Exercise, as simple as a brisk walking program, has been found to reduce the incidence of heart attack in 40- to 60-year-old women (Manson et al. 1999). In this study of female nurses (thus the name Nurses' Health Study), participants reported physical activity and exercise levels as well as heart disease that had developed over the course of eight years. The researchers indicate their findings "lend further support to current federal exercise guidelines, which endorse moderate-intensity exercise for at least 30 minutes on most (preferably all) days of the week. [The] results suggest that such a regimen (e.g., brisk walking for three or more hours per week) could reduce the risk of coronary events [heart attacks] in women by 30 to 40 percent. Increasing walking time or combining walking with vigorous exercise appears to be associated with even greater risk reductions" (Manson et al. 1999, 656). Additional research confirmed the benefits of walking and vigorous exercise and, in addition, clearly identified the increased cardiovascular risk for prolonged sitting (Manson et al. 2002). Therefore, it is definitely important for women to get up and get moving.

Maintaining a regular exercise program can also help combat obesity, one of the risk factors for cardiovascular disease. Increased body weight, often seen around the time of menopause, can be slowed or reversed with activity. Unfortunately, at the same time, muscle mass declines with age (American

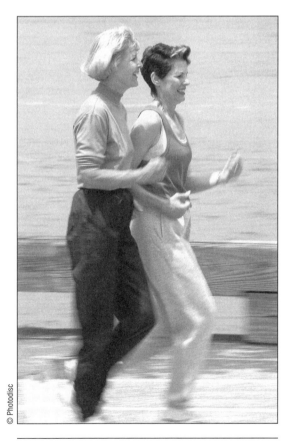

© Photodisc

Regular exercise provides many health benefits, helping you to feel more vibrant and energetic.

College of Sports Medicine [ACSM] 1998a). Strength training (as discussed in chapter 4) can provide you with a boost because muscle tissue is more metabolically active, which simply means that at rest you burn more calories. According to an American College of Sports Medicine (ACSM) position stand, strength training is "an effective way to increase energy requirements, decrease body fat mass, and maintain metabolically active tissue mass" (1998a, 996).

Aerobic exercise is also part of the big picture of maintaining a healthy body weight. Additionally, aerobic exercise is valuable in fighting other risk factors for heart disease. Individual responses will vary, but potential benefits include favorable changes in cholesterol levels (increasing the "good," or HDL, cholesterol and decreasing the "bad," or LDL, cholesterol) as well as triglycerides (Brubaker, Kaminsky, and Whaley 2002). As an additional benefit, aerobic exercise has been reported to reduce blood pressure in those with hypertension, although the amount of change observed appears to be quite individual and potentially based on preexercise blood pressure (Brubaker, Kaminsky, and Whaley 2002).

Although some cardiovascular risk factors are out of your control (e.g., family history or age), many can be controlled (e.g., smoking) or can be modified with lifestyle changes (e.g., body weight). In the Nurses' Health Study, women who did not smoke cigarettes, consumed alcohol moderately, were not overweight, had a healthy diet, and exercised moderately or vigorously 30 minutes each day had an 80 percent lower incidence of coronary heart disease than the rest of the population (Stampfer et al. 2000). Lifestyle modifications are effective. The exercise programs outlined in this book provide you with specific guidance in establishing a complete exercise plan.

Promotes Bone Health

Osteoporosis is a "skeletal disorder characterized by compromised bone strength predisposing to an increased risk of fracture" (Osteoporosis Prevention, Diagnosis, and Therapy 2001, 786), and it affects more women than men (NIH 2002). Diagnosis of osteoporosis may include measurement of bone density by DEXA (which stands for dual energy X-ray absorptiometry) or computed tomography (NIH 2002). Both of these tests provide a noninvasive analysis of the bone. In a review of osteoporosis completed by a group of researchers from around the globe, the suggestion was made that "severe bone loss and fractures are not natural consequences of aging but may be prevented or substantially delayed" (NIH 2002, 182). Peak bone mass occurs in the third decade and remains relatively stable in healthy women until menopause (NIH 2002; Osteoporosis Prevention, Diagnosis, and Therapy 2001). More specifically, bone mass is lost at a rate of .75 to 1 percent per year after a woman reaches the age of 35, but that rate increases to 2 to 3 percent per year at menopause (Burghardt 1999). The importance of optimizing bone mass before menopause is obvious—and exercise plays a vital, although not solo, role.

At menopause, estrogen levels decrease. The rapid bone loss seen at menopause is distinct from age-related losses (ACSM 2004). Decreased estrogen is thought to cause bone loss (ACSM 2004), although how this occurs has not been completely identified (NIH 2002). Of course, other factors that increase the likelihood of falling and fracture also come into the picture. These risks include cigarette smoking, low body weight, previous fracture, and family history of fracture (NIH 2002), as well as reduced muscle strength, reduced flexibility in the lower body, and reduced postural control (ACSM 2004). Physical activity is therefore a key component in prevention of fracture. In the Nurses' Health Study, the relative risk of hip fracture decreased by six percent for every additional hour of walking per week (ACSM 2004). Even though the benefits on bone mineral density may be minimal, lower-intensity weight-bearing exercise like walking provides potential benefits.

Guidelines to reduce the risk of osteoporosis are important for all adults but women in particular because of the higher prevalence of osteoporosis. Recommendations by an international panel of researchers (NIH 2002) include the following advice:

- Avoid tobacco use.
- Drink alcohol in moderation, if at all.
- Consume adequate calcium and vitamin D (see chapter 7 for more information). Calcium and exercise may have a synergistic effect—in other words, the combination is of greater benefit than just adding the benefits of each separately.
- Undertake a reasonable program of physical activity.

Physical activity that benefits bone is not necessarily the same activity that benefits the cardiorespiratory system. It appears that to improve bone density, weight-bearing activity such as jogging, jumping, and calisthenics (Nelson and Sequin 2004) is best. In addition, progressive resistance training, or weight training, can provide the needed stress to stimulate the bone (see chapter 4). "As muscles lift a particular load, they pull against tendons, which thereby exert that force on bone, causing bone growth" (Nelson and Sequin 2004, 95). When loads are placed on bone, bone mass is increased, and the converse is true as well (Marcus 2001). Again, you should avoid inactivity.

Recent research has specifically focused on postmenopausal women. During one study, researchers asked postmenopausal women between the ages of 40 and 65 to follow a three-day-per-week program of stretching, balance, weightlifting, and some moderate-impact activities (e.g., walking, jogging, skipping, hopping). After one year, the women's bone mineral density (i.e., bone strength) was improved (Cussler et al. 2003). A previous study demonstrated the benefits of two days per week of relatively high-intensity strength training, which allowed a group of postmenopausal women (ages 50-70 years) to preserve bone density as well as improve muscle mass, strength, and balance over a one-year period (Nelson et al. 1994). Incorporating physical activity into your schedule benefits your bones as well as the rest of your body systems. ACSM's position stand notes "physical activities that help preserve muscle mass (e.g., resistance exercise) may also be effective in preserving bone mass" (ACSM 2004, 1990).

For some women, drug therapy may be appropriate. Exercise alone cannot prevent all bone loss during postmenopause (Drinkwater 1999, ACSM 2004). Many medications are available for women including estrogen therapy, selective estrogen receptor modulator (SERM) therapy (e.g., raloxifene), and bisphosphonates (e.g., alendronate, risedronate) among some others. The decision of which, if any, medication is appropriate should be made in conjunction with a physician, in light of individual health situations. For more information on medications, see the sidebar on page 16.

Even though medications may be needed, one should not rule out exercise as part of the picture. Strength training increases muscle mass and strength along with dynamic balance (ACSM 1998a). The sum total of benefits may reduce the risk of fracture. Although drug therapy plays a potential role, "traditional pharmacological and nutritional approaches to the treatment or prevention of osteoporosis have the capacity to maintain or slow the loss of bone but not the ability to improve balance, strength, muscle mass, or physical activity" (ACSM 1998a, 996). This concept is supported by the Erlangen Fitness Osteoporosis Prevention Study (EFOPS) done in Germany involving women with some impairment in bone density (osteopenia). In that study, early postmenopausal women between the ages of 48 and 60 years (corresponding to 1-8 years postmenopause) exercised four times each week, including endurance training, jumping, strength training, and stretching. Outcomes after one year included positive findings not only for bone mineral density of the lower spine but also for insomnia, mood, life satisfaction, strength, and endurance (Kemmler et al. 2002). EFOPS continued for another year, and at the two-year mark the exercising women still had significantly better strength and endurance, less bone loss and back pain, and lower cholesterol and triglycerides than nonexercising women (Kemmler et al. 2004). The case for an active lifestyle and complete exercise plan for the long term is clearly supported.

Drug Therapy for Bone Health

Hormone therapy (estrogen only or combined estrogen and progestin) has been shown to offer protection against fracture (Banks et al. 2004). Protective effects on bone appear shortly after the initiation of hormone therapy but also unfortunately are short-lived after use ceases (Banks et al. 2004). For more information on other health benefits and risks associated with hormone therapy, see the sidebar on page 8.

Selective estrogen receptor modulators (SERMs) are an alternative to the traditional hormone therapy (HT). Raloxifene has been approved for both prevention and treatment of osteoporosis (Wilson 2003). It differs from traditional HT because it works on the bone to provide estrogen's benefits without the unwanted action on the breast (i.e., breast cancer) or endometrium (i.e., uterine cancer). Raloxifene has also been found to lower cholesterol (total and LDL) levels as well as increase bone mineral density (Delmas et al. 1997). Risk factors with raloxifene therapy include increased risk of thromboembolic disease (Purdie 1999), although the risk appears confined to the first several months of therapy (Draper 2003). Thromboembolic disease involves a thrombus, or clot, moving through the bloodstream and becoming lodged in a blood vessel, causing a blockage. The benefits of HT therapy on hot flashes are not found with raloxifene, and actually, in some cases hot flashes may be increased (Wilson 2003). Research is still underway to examine the effectiveness of this medication.

Bisphosphonates are drugs that inhibit bone breakdown. Risedronate and alendronate sodium are approved by the FDA for both prevention and treatment of osteoporosis. Risedronate has been found to reduce fractures of the spine as well as other fractures (McClung 2003). Alendronate appears to have benefits for both younger and older postmenopausal women (McClung 2003). Taking bisphosphonates with or after meals limits the absorption of these drugs (McClung 2003). Potential side effects of bisphosphonates include gastrointestinal problems and irritation of the esophagus (inflammation or ulcers).

Discussion of your specific health situation with your health care provider is vital. Each woman has a unique situation that must be considered individually. General recommendations discussed in this chapter include calcium and vitamin D intake, avoiding certain risk factors (e.g., smoking), and incorporating regular physical activity into your life. The inclusion of various drug or hormone therapies will depend on your personal health history and medical conditions; you should carefully discuss these with your physician.

Prevents Depression

Depression or depressive symptoms are found in about 15 percent of older adults (ACSM 1998a). A number of studies conducted over many years (i.e., longitudinal studies, which continuously examine a group of individuals over an extended time period) seem to indicate some benefit of exercise on depressive symptoms, although the reason for this positive influence is not known at this time (ACSM 1998a). Physical activity has also been found to influence self-efficacy, or one's perception of control (ACSM 1998a).

Reduces Breast Cancer Risk

Physical activity appears to provide some protective effects against breast cancer. One study that tracked more than 25,000 women for 13 years found evidence that physical activity during leisure time and at work was associated with a reduced breast cancer risk (Thune et al. 1997). The reason for this decline may include the avoidance of obesity—in particular gynoid obesity (i.e., fat accumulation around the waist) (Nieman 1999). The reduction of body fat resulting from a regular physical activity program may be one of the main means by which exercise can influence breast cancer risk (Thune et al. 1997). Other contributing factors associated with exercise include the reduction of some hormones by strenuous exercise, increased energy expenditure, changes in insulin (higher blood insulin promotes the growth of breast cancer cells), and enhancement of the body's own immune system (Nieman 1999).

In another recent study, regular physical activity was associated with a lower risk of breast cancer (McTiernan et al. 2003). Moderate physical activity (e.g., walking, biking outdoors, easy swimming, popular or folk dancing) as well as more vigorous activity (e.g., jogging, tennis, swimming laps, aerobics, aerobic dancing) were reviewed in a group of 74,171 women between the ages of 50 and 79 years. The study included consideration of past exercise as well as current activity levels. Specifically, women who had engaged in regular strenuous physical activity when they were age 35 had a 14 percent decreased risk of breast cancer. When considering the current physical activity of the women in this study, researchers found women with the greatest total activity scores had the greatest reduction in breast cancer risk. The scores for total activity were a composite of the frequency and duration of exercise in addition to the intensity level. The higher this score was, the greater the reduction in breast cancer risk (up to a 21 percent reduction in the most active group) (McTiernan et al. 2003). It appears that engaging in moderate to vigorous physical activity for 45 minutes or more on five or more days per week is sufficient to confer a reduced risk of not only breast cancer but also colon cancer (Byers et al. 2002), although researchers have not definitively found the ideal exercise level (McTiernan et al. 2003).

Cancer survivors benefit from physical activity as well. Exercise has been reported to improve or alleviate the following conditions in breast cancer survivors (Brown et al. 2003):

- Cardiorespiratory fitness
- Muscle strength
- Body composition
- Fatigue
- Anxiety
- Depression
- Self-esteem
- Happiness

Each of the listed improvement areas provides for a combined improvement in quality of life—including physical benefits as well as functional and emotional benefits (Brown et al. 2003). Whether physical activity can reduce the chance of cancer reoccurrence is not known (American Cancer Society 2003).

Summary

Menopause may be the end of your monthly menstrual cycle, but this time in your life can be one of new beginnings as well. Your selection of this book is evidence that you are an action-oriented woman. Take special note of the action plan check-offs at the conclusion of each chapter. Our focus in this book is to equip you with the information and resources needed to develop an effective and complete personalized exercise plan—and to fit that plan into your life. Let's get started!

ACTION PLAN:

THRIVING WITH HORMONAL CHANGES

- ☐ Understand the timing of menopause and the related hormonal changes.
- ☐ Consult with your physician regarding changes in menstrual bleeding.
- ☐ Examine how you can most effectively deal with hot flashes.
- ☐ Develop a regular sleep routine.
- ☐ Consult with your physician regarding hormone therapy to determine if it is appropriate for you.

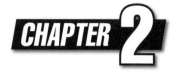

FINDING THE RIGHT EXERCISE FIT

Exercise is simply one of the best things you can do for yourself. Often the effects of the aging process are mixed or, more accurately, confounded by an increasingly inactive lifestyle. According to the National Institute on Aging, "Together, lack of exercise and poor diet are the second-largest underlying cause of death in the United States. (Smoking is the #1 cause.)" (National Institute on Aging 2001, 4).

In this chapter we review basic concepts of exercise as well as identify the three main components of a balanced exercise program. Your exercise program must be based on your needs, current health status, and goals. The practical aspects of developing your personal exercise program are discussed. Specific recommendations for your exercise program are fully defined in chapters 3, 4, and 5.

Physical Activity Versus Exercise

Physical activity and exercise—are they the same or different? Actually, exercise is simply a specific type of physical activity that focuses on physical fitness. Let's consider some definitions and then we will discuss the focus of this book.

Physical activity is any movement that involves effort and so burns calories (ACSM 2000). It includes everything from gardening to washing the car to vacuuming the floor. It also includes a planned exercise program.

Exercise is a more focused, or specific, aspect of physical activity (ACSM 2000). The concept of movement and effort is the same, but the goal is to improve physical fitness rather than to simply accomplish day-to-day task-related activities. The components of physical fitness are cardiorespiratory endurance, muscle strength and endurance, and flexibility. Each of these building blocks are described later in this chapter.

Physically fit people are those who can complete activities of daily living as well as planned exercise without limitations caused by lack of endurance, strength, or flexibility (ACSM 2000). By maintaining an exercise program that includes these three fitness components, you will more easily be able to accomplish other activities during the course of the day. For example, we (the authors) both enjoy working in our yards, and in doing so, plant trees, water plants, and mow the grass (with push mowers!). Each of these tasks is made easier by the fitness gained in our exercise programs. Lifting, reaching, and repetitive movements, which occur during routine yard maintenance, could produce major physical stress without a solid foundation of fitness. Part of the purpose of this book is to provide you with an action plan to progress toward becoming physically fit or to maintain the fitness you have already achieved as you move into menopause. You will benefit from building or maintaining your fitness foundation every day, in each physical activity in which you participate.

The Surgeon General's Report on Physical Activity and Health was released in 1996; you may remember some television or print coverage of the report. Within this comprehensive report, which included input from many organizations, a number of specific health benefits were listed (see the sidebar on page 21). The report also documents health benefits of physical activity and includes the following findings (U.S. Department of Health and Human Services [US DHHS] 1996):

- People who are usually inactive can improve their health and well-being by becoming even moderately active on a regular basis.
- Physical activity need not be strenuous to give you health benefits.
- You can achieve greater health benefits by increasing the amount (duration, frequency, or intensity) of physical activity.

The first and second bullet points relate to physical activity. The Surgeon General's report emphasizes the health benefits of including "a moderate amount of physical activity . . . on most, if not all, days of the week" (US DHHS 1996). Our focus in this book concerns exercise recommendations alluded to in the third bullet. Specifically, the report states the following: "Additional health benefits can be gained through greater amounts of physical activity. People who can maintain a regular regimen of activity that is of greater duration or of more vigorous intensity are likely to derive greater benefit" (US DHHS 1996). This regular regimen falls under our definition of exercise. Such regular, planned, structured activity (that is, exercise) is the focus of this book.

Health Benefits of Exercise

Regular physical activity that is performed on most days of the week reduces the risk of developing or dying from some of the leading causes of illness and death in the United States. Regular physical activity improves health in the following ways:

- Reduces the risk of dying prematurely.
- Reduces the risk of dying from heart disease.
- Reduces the risk of developing diabetes.
- Reduces the risk of developing high blood pressure.
- Helps reduce blood pressure in people who already have high blood pressure.
- Reduces the risk of developing colon cancer.
- Reduces feelings of depression and anxiety.
- Helps control weight.
- Helps build and maintain healthy bones, muscles, and joints.
- Helps older adults become stronger and better able to move about without falling.
- Promotes psychological well-being.

US Department of Health and Human Services (US DHHS), 1996. "Physical Activity and Health: A Report of the Surgeon General" (Atlanta: Centers for Disease Control and Prevention, National Center for Chronic Disease Prevention and Health Promotion).

Components of an Exercise Program

A solid exercise program is like a sturdy three-legged chair. If one leg is weak, the chair isn't stable. In the same way, ignoring one of the exercise components can put your fitness program out of balance. Each component—cardiorespiratory endurance, muscular fitness, and flexibility—is important and must be considered.

Cardiorespiratory Endurance

Cardiorespiratory endurance is the ability to perform large-muscle, repetitive, moderate- to high-intensity exercise for extended periods of time (ACSM 2000). Brisk walking for 30 minutes is an example of a cardiorespiratory endurance activity.

The importance of cardiorespiratory fitness cannot be ignored. With good cardiorespiratory fitness you can avoid dying prematurely, especially as related to heart disease, and you will have the capability to be more active in all parts of your life—which has additional health benefits as well (ACSM 2000). Chapter 3 explains in detail how to determine your current cardiorespiratory fitness level as well as how to select activities to improve in this area.

Muscular Fitness

Muscular fitness is a general term that incorporates both muscular strength and muscular endurance. Strength and endurance are two ends of the muscle fitness continuum. On one end is muscular strength, defined as the force the muscle can generate in one maximal effort. An example of muscular strength is the ability to lift a heavy chair when rearranging a room. Without sufficient muscular strength, you would be unable to move the chair. On the other end of the continuum is muscular endurance, defined as the ability of a muscle to make repeated contractions or to sustain a contraction. An example would be holding a heavy bag of groceries—you must sustain the contraction or watch your produce roll down the street.

The importance of muscular fitness is also well established. Muscular fitness maintains or improves the following (ACSM 2000):

- Muscle mass, which boosts metabolic rate (muscle burns more calories than does fat tissue in the body) and is related to body weight
- Bone mass, which is related to bone strength (or conversely osteoporosis)
- Muscle–tendon integrity, which is related to lower injury risk
- Ability to carry out activities of daily living

Muscular fitness is vital for women, especially as they age. Big, bulging muscles are not needed for improvements in strength, but toned muscles will benefit you in your routine physical activities at work and home as well as during recreational activities. Many women have little exposure to, or experience with, resistance training and thus have avoided it. In chapter 4, we remove the mystique and provide you with the background to create a simple and effective strength program. By incorporating resistance training exercises, as described in chapter 4, you can supercharge your fitness program.

Flexibility

Flexibility involves the ability to move a joint or joints through a range of motion and the related capability to complete specific tasks (ACSM 1998a). Flexibility allows you to carry out daily activities as well as movements associated with exercise. The range of motion you have is joint-specific. This means a person may have good flexibility at the shoulder joint but below-average flexibility at the hip. The benefits of performing stretching activities include the following (ACSM 1998b):

- Improved joint range of motion
- Improved joint function
- Enhanced muscular performance

Each of these benefits becomes especially important as women age. The aging process results in loss of flexibility in tendons (connective tissue that attaches muscle to bone) as well as decrease in the range of motion. To combat the changes caused by aging, you should include a stretching program to complete the exercise prescription. Chapter 5 describes stretching activities that you can use to maintain or improve your flexibility.

Exercise Principles

The effectiveness of your exercise training program depends on your body's response to the activities you select. Physiology is the study of how the body works. The physiological principles that apply to a training program include overload, specificity, progression, and maintenance.

Overload

The term *overload* simply means the activity in which you are engaging is beyond the normal level of exertion of that muscle or body system. The principle of overload is often applied to strength training. For example, to build a stronger muscle, a person must stress that muscle by lifting a weight heavier than she typically lifts. Lifting a pencil from your desk 10 times will not stress your muscles. However, lifting a 10-pound dumbbell 10 times may be an overload. The emphasis is on going beyond what the muscle is normally accustomed to doing.

Although commonly used with strength training, the concept of overload is also appropriately applied to cardiorespiratory training. By exercising at higher intensity or longer duration, you can provide a unique stress on the cardiorespiratory system (including the heart and lungs). When faced with a higher demand, the body's response will be to change (i.e., improve) to meet that demand. This is a positive training adaptation. Thus, both muscles and the cardiorespiratory system can adapt, or change, to meet increased demands. The process by which those changes occur is overload.

Specificity

Specificity refers to adaptations specific to the exercise you do as well as the muscles involved (ACSM 2000). These adaptations occur in both metabolic and physiological functioning (McArdle, Katch, and Katch 2001). Metabolic function deals with changes in the cells of the body—in particular, how they break down food for fuel. For example, a marathon runner prepares for a marathon by running for long durations for months before the actual race. This stress on the body will allow her to better burn fat for energy (which is very economical) because her body has learned to adapt to long-duration activity. The same adaptation would not result from walking slowly for 10 minutes each day. The adaptation observed is very specific to the type of stress placed on the body.

Specificity also deals with physiological functions—that is, with how the body works and how the body adapts to increased work. Physiologically, the marathoner just described will also show improved blood flow to her muscles. This allows her to have more oxygen available to the working muscles, which will make the long-duration activity easier for her. The training for a marathon will not, however, improve her 100-yard dash. The marathon is an endurance event, and the 100-yard dash is a sprint, or anaerobic, event that does not rely on oxygen delivery to the muscles. The adaptations are specific to the training. Similarly, if you were to start lifting a 10-pound bag of flour with your right arm, your right arm would become stronger. However, if no stress were placed on your left arm, the left arm would remain unchanged. To elicit a change, the specific muscle group must experience the increase in work.

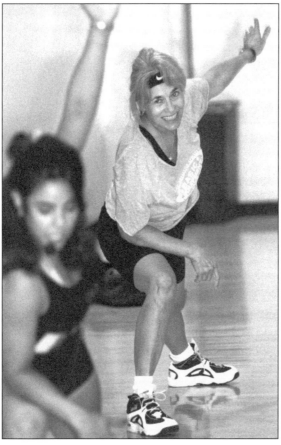

© davidsandersphotos.com

The benefits you derive from exercise are specific to the kind of exercise you do.

Progression

The principle of progression suggests that you must periodically increase the workload in order for it to actually remain an overload. As your body adapts to an initial workload, it will become easier for you, and therefore not much of an overload. For example, a woman starts a weightlifting program and initially lifts a five-pound weight for 10 repetitions. After doing this exercise for a month, lifting the five-pound weight 10 times might be quite easy—in other words, the muscles have adapted and become stronger. To continue to see improvements, the woman would need to increase the weight lifted.

Note that progression needs to be gradual to allow the body to make adaptations to a given overload before increasing the workload. Charting your progress by recording your workouts is a good way to determine where you may need to make changes. For strength training, progression may involve increasing the number of repetitions or increasing the amount of weight lifted. For cardiorespiratory training, progression could involve increasing the intensity of the exercise (e.g., walking more briskly) or increasing the length of the workout (e.g., walking for 40 minutes rather than 30 minutes).

Maintenance and Reversibility

Any gains made can be lost if you cease the activity. If you stop your resistance training program, you will lose strength. If you stop your walking program, you will lose cardiorespiratory benefits. If you stop stretching, you will lose flexibility. Each component of your exercise program is a "use it or lose it" phenomenon. Unfortunately, all the benefits that can be gained are reversible and can be diminished if neglected. For example, one research study documented that cardiorespiratory fitness was significantly reduced after only two weeks of no training (ACSM 1998b). Maintaining the benefits of your exercise program (to be described in the next section) requires you to regularly participate in appropriate activities.

Developing Your Exercise Program

Before beginning an exercise program, it is recommended that you complete a simple health appraisal to determine if there is any reason you should see your physician before starting. A very common self-administered questionnaire is the Physical Activity Readiness Questionnaire (PAR-Q). Take a moment to complete the PAR-Q, which is in figure 2.1. If you honestly answer yes to any of the questions, a visit to your physician would be recommended before you start any exercise program.

The intent of this book is to help you develop an efficient and effective workout program. Having a good plan is fine, but implementing that plan on a consistent, regular basis is the only way to realize the benefits. The likelihood of your exercise program being workable in your life depends on your consideration of timing, frequency, and location.

Physical Activity Readiness
Questionnaire - PAR-Q
(revised 2002)

PAR-Q & YOU

(A Questionnaire for People Aged 15 to 69)

Regular physical activity is fun and healthy, and increasingly more people are starting to become more active every day. Being more active is very safe for most people. However, some people should check with their doctor before they start becoming much more physically active.

If you are planning to become much more physically active than you are now, start by answering the seven questions in the box below. If you are between the ages of 15 and 69, the PAR-Q will tell you if you should check with your doctor before you start. If you are over 69 years of age, and you are not used to being very active, check with your doctor.

Common sense is your best guide when you answer these questions. Please read the questions carefully and answer each one honestly: check YES or NO.

YES	NO		
☐	☐	1.	Has your doctor ever said that you have a heart condition <u>and</u> that you should only do physical activity recommended by a doctor?
☐	☐	2.	Do you feel pain in your chest when you do physical activity?
☐	☐	3.	In the past month, have you had chest pain when you were not doing physical activity?
☐	☐	4.	Do you lose your balance because of dizziness or do you ever lose consciousness?
☐	☐	5.	Do you have a bone or joint problem (for example, back, knee or hip) that could be made worse by a change in your physical activity?
☐	☐	6.	Is your doctor currently prescribing drugs (for example, water pills) for your blood pressure or heart condition?
☐	☐	7.	Do you know of <u>any other reason</u> why you should not do physical activity?

If

you

answered

YES to one or more questions

Talk with your doctor by phone or in person BEFORE you start becoming much more physically active or BEFORE you have a fitness appraisal. Tell your doctor about the PAR-Q and which questions you answered YES.

• You may be able to do any activity you want — as long as you start slowly and build up gradually. Or, you may need to restrict your activities to those which are safe for you. Talk with your doctor about the kinds of activities you wish to participate in and follow his/her advice.

• Find out which community programs are safe and helpful for you.

NO to all questions

If you answered NO honestly to <u>all</u> PAR-Q questions, you can be reasonably sure that you can:
• start becoming much more physically active – begin slowly and build up gradually. This is the safest and easiest way to go.

• take part in a fitness appraisal – this is an excellent way to determine your basic fitness so that you can plan the best way for you to live actively. It is also highly recommended that you have your blood pressure evaluated. If your reading is over 144/94, talk with your doctor before you start becoming much more physically active.

DELAY BECOMING MUCH MORE ACTIVE:
• if you are not feeling well because of a temporary illness such as a cold or a fever – wait until you feel better; or

• if you are or may be pregnant – talk to your doctor before you start becoming more active.

PLEASE NOTE: If your health changes so that you then answer YES to any of the above questions, tell your fitness or health professional. Ask whether you should change your physical activity plan.

<u>Informed Use of the PAR-Q</u>: The Canadian Society for Exercise Physiology, Health Canada, and their agents assume no liability for persons who undertake physical activity, and if in doubt after completing this questionnaire, consult your doctor prior to physical activity.

No changes permitted. You are encouraged to photocopy the PAR-Q but only if you use the entire form.

NOTE: If the PAR-Q is being given to a person before he or she participates in a physical activity program or a fitness appraisal, this section may be used for legal or administrative purposes.

"I have read, understood and completed this questionnaire. Any questions I had were answered to my full satisfaction."

NAME _____

SIGNATURE _____ DATE _____

SIGNATURE OF PARENT _____ WITNESS _____
or GUARDIAN (for participants under the age of majority)

Note: This physical activity clearance is valid for a maximum of 12 months from the date it is completed and becomes invalid if your condition changes so that you would answer YES to any of the seven questions.

CSEP
SCPE © Canadian Society for Exercise Physiology   Supported by: [🍁] Health Santé
Canada Canada

continued on other side…

Figure 2.1 Physical Activity Readiness Questionnaire (PAR-Q).
From *Action Plan for Menopause* by Barbara Bushman and Janice Clark Young, 2005, Champaign, IL: Human Kinetics.

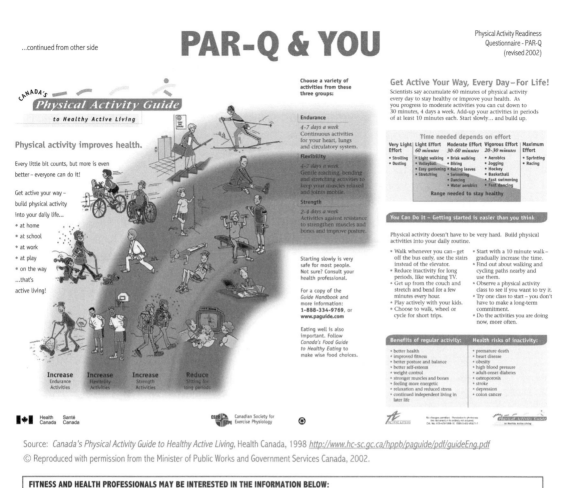

PAR-Q & YOU

...continued from other side

Physical Activity Readiness
Questionnaire - PAR-Q
(revised 2002)

Source: *Canada's Physical Activity Guide to Healthy Active Living*, Health Canada, 1998 http://www.hc-sc.gc.ca/hppb/paguide/pdf/guideEng.pdf

© Reproduced with permission from the Minister of Public Works and Government Services Canada, 2002.

FITNESS AND HEALTH PROFESSIONALS MAY BE INTERESTED IN THE INFORMATION BELOW:

The following companion forms are available for doctors' use by contacting the Canadian Society for Exercise Physiology (address below):

The **Physical Activity Readiness Medical Examination (PARmed-X)** – to be used by doctors with people who answer YES to one or more questions on the PAR-Q.

The **Physical Activity Readiness Medical Examination for Pregnancy (PARmed-X for Pregnancy)** – to be used by doctors with pregnant patients who wish to become more active.

References:

Arraix, G.A., Wigle, D.T., Mao, Y. (1992). Risk Assessment of Physical Activity and Physical Fitness in the Canada Health Survey Follow-Up Study. **J. Clin. Epidemiol.** 45:4 419-428.

Mottola, M., Wolfe, L.A. (1994). Active Living and Pregnancy, In: A. Quinney, L. Gauvin, T. Wall (eds.), **Toward Active Living: Proceedings of the International Conference on Physical Activity, Fitness and Health**. Champaign, IL: Human Kinetics.

PAR-Q Validation Report, British Columbia Ministry of Health, 1978.

Thomas, S., Reading, J., Shephard, R.J. (1992). Revision of the Physical Activity Readiness Questionnaire (PAR-Q). **Can. J. Spt. Sci.** 17:4 338-345.

To order multiple printed copies of the PAR-Q, please contact the:

Canadian Society for Exercise Physiology
202-185 Somerset Street West
Ottawa, ON K2P 0J2
Tel. 1-877-651-3755 • FAX (613) 234-3565
Online: www.csep.ca

The original PAR-Q was developed by the British Columbia Ministry of Health. It has been revised by an Expert Advisory Committee of the Canadian Society for Exercise Physiology chaired by Dr. N. Gledhill (2002).

Disponible en français sous le titre «Questionnaire sur l'aptitude à l'activité physique - Q-AAP (revisé 2002)».

 © Canadian Society for Exercise Physiology   Supported by:  Health Canada   Santé Canada

From *Action Plan for Menopause* by Barbara Bushman and Janice Clark Young, 2005, Champaign, IL: Human Kinetics.

Source: Physical Activity Readiness Questionnaire (PAR-Q) © 2002. Reprinted with permission from the Canadian Society for Exercise Physiology. http://www.csep.ca/forms.asp

Timing

Time crunches, unfinished to-do lists, endless responsibilities—how does a woman find time in a busy day to include exercise? We recommend you make it a number one priority. Does that sound too simple? If so, that is good! Exercise *is* pretty simple, though we often make it complex. Chapters 3, 4, and 5 explain the three components of fitness (cardiorespiratory exercise, muscular fitness, and flexibility) so you will feel confident in the activities you select. But, how do you find time to include physical activity and exercise in your life? We have some suggestions.

Pull out your calendar, daily planner, or computerized schedule (yes, we really mean it). Note that your calendar holds the same number of days per week and hours per day as everyone else's. Now, consider the importance of an exercise program to your health and well-being. We have pointed out benefits to your heart and your bones as well as to menopausal symptom and disease reduction. Are you ready now to schedule exercise on your calendar, just as you would any important appointment?

Making your workout a priority is one of the first steps to making exercise a lifelong habit. The actual time of day you choose isn't as important as ensuring time is set aside. Some women find a morning routine is a great way to kick-start the day. Others prefer to exercise over the lunch hour and use the midday workout to recharge for the afternoon. Still others enjoy exercising later in the day. There is no magic formula—simply find a time that works for you and stick with it. Look at your calendar, find time slots, schedule time for exercise, and keep those appointments.

Second, develop a plan. What are your goals? Are you plagued by hot flashes? Are you concerned about your body weight? Do you wish you could keep pace with your spouse, kids, or grandkids? Baseline recommendations for overall health include a cardiorespiratory component (termed aerobic exercise), a muscular fitness component, and a flexibility component. Whether you intend to begin an exercise program for the first time or you are looking for hints to continue successfully, you must have a plan. Details given in the next three chapters will help you develop a specific exercise prescription.

Frequency

You will want to include three or four days per week of aerobic training (cardiorespiratory system workout, such as walking or jogging—see chapter 3 for specifics) as well as two or three days for muscular fitness (see chapter 4 for more details). A flexibility program can be incorporated on one of the other training days, or you may find it a relaxing close to your day (see chapter 5 for some great recommendations). If you are just starting a program you may want to consider scheduling some exercise time every other day. This will help you establish a routine. If your goals include weight loss or even competitive goals (e.g., a local 5K run), you may want to consider building up to five or six days per week.

Location

Location, location, location. That is the real estate mantra. When it comes to exercise, there is no need for fancy equipment—although using equipment is great, too. You do not need to join a health club—although the exercise options available at many facilities are also nice. You need to determine what is best for you. Location is often tied to time. Finding time to drive to a fitness facility may be difficult, or perhaps you don't want to pay a membership fee. If so, don't give up—be creative at home.

You can develop a wonderful exercise program to do in your home and your neighborhood by looking around. Do you live in an area where you can walk safely on sidewalks or along the road (remember to always face traffic)? If so, you can start a walking or jogging program. Do you have some old milk jugs? If so, you can fill them with varying amounts of water to provide resistance for strength training. Purchasing some large elastic resistance bands can allow you to do many resistance training activities in your home. Stretching activities can be done almost anywhere and are a great at-home exercise. Chapter 8 includes additional information on purchasing home exercise equipment, as well as pointers on what to look for in a health club.

Putting Goals on Paper

Setting goals—both long term and short term—is an important step. Although we strongly believe in the importance of all three legs of the "exercise chair" (cardiorespiratory endurance, muscular fitness, and flexibility), you need to approach these recommendations from your own perspective. For goals to be met, they must be measurable. Long-term goals include those to be achieved in the future, maybe six months or a year from now. Short-term goals include weekly and monthly goals. As you establish short-term goals, be sure they ultimately lead you to achievement of your long-term goals.

Short-Term Goals

Short-term goals are those that can realistically be achieved within a brief period of time. For example, if you have not been involved in any exercise before picking up this book, a short-term goal might be to walk 10 minutes around your neighborhood every day for a week. This is much better than stating a goal as "I will exercise more." Note that the latter statement is not measurable. The idea of exercising "more" is too ambiguous. The former statement is very specific and is realistically achievable. As you meet one set of short-term goals, you should set new goals. This follows the principle of progression.

Writing down your goals is helpful. Some women put their exercise goals in their daily planners or on a chart on the refrigerator. By keeping your short-term goals prominent, you are reminded to continue and thus will be encouraged. Checking off completed goals helps you stay on course. It is important to note that these are *your* goals. Self-imposed goals are so much better than those imposed by others. Your exercise program belongs to *you*.

Long-Term Goals

Long-term goals are those fitness points you plan to achieve in the future. It is still important to keep these goals realistic and measurable. For example, if you are just starting an exercise program, you might set a long-term goal of participating in a community event such as a 5K walk (note: 5 kilometers is 3.1 miles). This would be an inappropriate goal for one month from now because it would not be realistically achievable and may seem overwhelming. It is, however, a great goal for the future. Short-term goals of increasing walking time will ultimately lead to achieving the long-term goal.

Setting goals in each of the fitness areas we have discussed (cardiorespiratory, muscular, flexibility) allows you to individualize your progress. You may have already been walking, but after reading chapter 4, you realize you have neglected the area of muscular strength and endurance. By creating specific goals for each component of fitness, the outcome will give you a complete fitness perspective. (See the worksheet for exercise goals in chapter 8.)

Rewarding Yourself

Achievement of goals, short term or long term, is a reason to celebrate. Rewarding yourself for attaining a goal is a means of positive reinforcement. For example, after a month of consistently walking each day, you may reward yourself with a new article of clothing to be worn while exercising. Rewards do not need to be tangible, however. Self-reinforcement can also take the form of increased self-esteem and enhanced confidence in your physical abilities. After establishing a firm fitness foundation, you may find it possible to do other activities you were unable to participate in previously because of lack of fitness. The authors both enjoy activities made easier by a solid fitness base, including ballroom dancing, open-water kayaking, windsurfing, hiking, and gardening. The ability to do these activities with ease and enjoyment is a function of a regular exercise program that includes cardiorespiratory and muscular conditioning as well as stretching for flexibility.

Dealing With Unachieved Goals

Although it would be wonderful, you will not meet every fitness goal within the time line established. Sickness, travel, family responsibilities, work obligations, and other unavoidable situations may interrupt your plans. Realize interruptions are just that—short-term setbacks that do not need to permanently derail your fitness program. Each season brings challenges. Wintertime often brings illness such as colds and flu, which requires a temporary cessation of exercise. Summer months potentially bring vacations and schedule changes. Having a return plan must be part of your overall exercise plan.

For each setback, realize that you will need to roll back your time line. Reestablishing your exercise program after an illness will require you to start back slowly. For example, if you progressed from 10 minutes a day to 30 minutes a day but then missed a week of exercise because of illness, you should not start exercising at 30 minutes per day. Depending on your illness, you may need to slide back to 10 minutes per day until you build back to your previous level. Rather than being discouraged, be encouraged that you are able to regain your fitness level.

You may also find that your priorities change. What initially appeared to be a realistic and desired goal may no longer be desired. Goals are what *you* make them to be and are under your control. Goals are helpful in charting a path but must be flexible in light of changing priorities or even changing health status.

Summary

Physical activity and exercise should be a part of every person's life, and this is particularly true for women during menopause. The benefits of exercise have been well documented. Including all three exercise components described in this chapter (cardiorespiratory endurance, muscular fitness, and flexibility) provides you with a balanced program. By writing down your goals, both short term and long term, you will develop a solid plan for the future. Over the next three chapters you will read details on how to develop your own personalized exercise program based on your current fitness level and your goals. And then in the following chapters, we provide commonsense information on nutrition and how to realistically put your exercise plan into action.

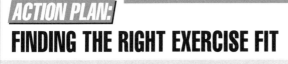

FINDING THE RIGHT EXERCISE FIT

- ☐ Consider the balance of cardiorespiratory endurance, muscular strength and endurance, and flexibility that you want to incorporate into your exercise program.
- ☐ Complete the Physical Activity Readiness Questionnaire (PAR-Q), and consult your physician if you honestly answer yes to any of the questions.
- ☐ Schedule time for exercise in your weekly schedule.
- ☐ Determine the best location for your exercise program.
- ☐ Write down your short-term and long-term fitness goals.

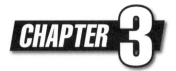

CHAPTER 3

INVIGORATING YOUR HEART HEALTH

The word *aerobic* means "with oxygen," and aerobic exercise includes those activities that make you breathe more heavily than you do at rest and also raise your heart rate. Cardiorespiratory fitness includes the functioning of your lungs, heart, and blood vessels. During aerobic exercise, your muscles use more oxygen; this requires your heart and lungs to work harder to meet that demand. This exertion on your body brings about positive adaptations, which build your cardiorespiratory fitness level.

Aerobic exercise includes walking, jogging, biking, swimming, and other activities that use large muscle groups in a repetitive manner for an extended period of time (20 minutes or more). Selection of an activity is not difficult, and there are many choices. Focus on selecting what you enjoy doing, and you should find it easy to fit into your day. Table 3.1 on page 37 includes a list of aerobic activities to help you get started.

Benefits of Aerobic Exercise

Health benefits are a major reason to include physical activity in your life. In 1996, the Surgeon General released a report on physical activity and health (US DHHS 1996). In this comprehensive review, a number of benefits associated with activity were outlined (see the sidebar on page 21 in chapter 2 for a list). Despite the publication of these benefits and media attention given to the inactivity of Americans, not much has changed. As you read this book, we hope you are ready to break from the inactivity rut (or continue to avoid the rut) and get moving. According to the Surgeon General's report, "Significant health benefits can be obtained by including a moderate amount of physical activity (e.g., 30 minutes of brisk walking) on most, if not all, days of the week. Through a modest increase in daily activity, most Americans can improve their health and quality of life. . . . Additional health benefits can be gained through greater amounts of physical activity. People who can maintain a regular regimen of activity that is of longer duration or of more vigorous intensity are likely to derive greater benefit" (US DHHS 1996). These statements clearly identify the importance of regular aerobic activity.

Physical activity encompasses a broad range of activities including washing your car or gardening, as well as aerobic exercise such as walking and running. The focus in this chapter is aerobic exercise. The health benefits of aerobic exercise—such as reducing risk of heart disease, hypertension, obesity, and diabetes—are not the only reasons to begin or maintain an exercise program. Exercise is especially valuable during menopause.

Hot flashes are experienced by up to 75 percent of women (Burghardt 1999). Research studies comparing groups of exercisers and nonexercisers have repeatedly shown the exercisers to have a lower incidence of hot flashes or less severe hot flashes (Burghart 1999). Additional information on hot flashes can be found in chapter 1.

Aerobic activity, in particular weight-bearing exercise, is a positive step toward healthy bones as well. The benefits start during the premenopausal years. Researchers have documented higher bone density (stronger bones) in menopausal women who did high-impact and moderate-impact activities in premenopausal years. Even walking, which is a low-impact activity, has been suggested to strengthen bones (Burghart 1999). More specific information on osteoporosis and bone health is found in chapters 1 and 7.

The benefits of developing and maintaining a regular aerobic exercise program include universal health benefits and also specific benefits for menopausal women. In this chapter, we walk you through the development of your aerobic fitness plan and explain how to select an activity, how to determine how hard you should exercise, and how to decide length and frequency of your exercise sessions.

Anatomy of an Aerobic Exercise Session

A typical aerobic exercise session should include a warm-up of 10 to 20 minutes, an endurance phase of 20 to 60 minutes, and a cool-down of 5 to 10 minutes. See figure 3.1 to visualize the three-part exercise session. The warm-up leads into the main focus of the workout, which we call the endurance phase. The cool-down follows the endurance phase and allows your body to return to preexercise levels. Each component is important for an effective and safe workout. This chapter discusses each of these components and how you should determine time and effort of each phase.

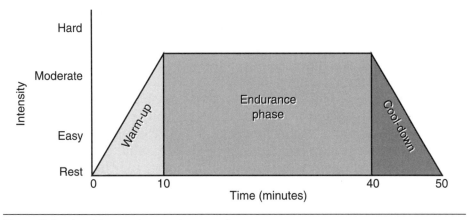

Figure 3.1 Aerobic exercise session overview.

Warm-Up

The warm-up includes 10 to 20 minutes of "transition" activities in which you are moving your body from rest to full preparation for the endurance phase of your workout. Consider the warm-up to be similar to an appetizer leading to a main course. A warm-up allows blood flow to increase to the muscles and prepares the body for the heightened demands of the endurance phase to come. The potential benefits of a warm-up include the following (ACSM 2000):

- Reduced susceptibility to injury
- Improved joint movements
- Enhanced muscular performance

The warm-up should be seen as a ramp into the endurance phase of the workout. Activities in a warm-up can include calisthenics and stretching (approximately 5-10 minutes) and low-intensity aerobic exercise (approximately 5-10 minutes). We recommend that you literally warm up, or increase your body temperature, with some easy aerobic activity, such as walking, before flexibility exercises (stretching). The reason is that "cold" muscles and body tissues are not as stretchable and are more likely to experience damage. By increasing body temperature before stretching, the benefits of the flexibility exercise can be achieved with lower risk for muscle or connective tissue damage (Nieman 1999). Details on stretching are covered in chapter 5.

The time spent warming up also depends on the intensity of the activity you plan to do in the endurance phase. If your target intensity is higher, it will take longer to make the transition to that workload. For example, if you will be jogging during the endurance phase, you will need to warm up longer than if your endurance activity includes walking. The higher the intensity level, the longer the warm-up needs to be. The goal is a smooth and easy transition. If your endurance phase includes fast walking, then the warm-up would include slower pace walking as well as some basic stretching. A warm-up should be individualized, and the time frame allotted can range from 10 minutes to prepare for a lower-intensity endurance phase and potentially up to 20 minutes for higher-intensity endurance phase exercise.

The key for an effective warm-up is to gradually prepare the body for the upcoming activity, starting out easy and building close to your target intensity for the endurance phase. You should avoid abruptly starting your workout—a warm-up is essential to prepare your heart, lungs, and muscles for the endurance phase of your exercise session.

Endurance Phase

If the warm-up is the appetizer, then the endurance phase is the main course. The real stimulus for cardiorespiratory conditioning occurs during this phase. The activities and how hard you do those activities (the intensity) determines your time frame. Typically, we prescribe 20 to 60 minutes. If you plan higher-intensity exercise, then target 20 minutes in the endurance phase. If you plan lower-intensity activity, then you would target a longer duration, potentially building up to 60 minutes. The balance between time and intensity is like a teeter-totter—when one is up then the other is down. For lower intensity, the time spent exercising will need to be greater; at a higher intensity, the time spent working out can be less.

You may be wondering which balance is best. There is no simple answer; an ideal workout for you depends on whether you are a beginner or an established exerciser, as well as your goals for your fitness program and your current health status. The prescription for the endurance phase of your workout will include manipulation of mode, intensity, duration, and frequency.

Selecting an Enjoyable Exercise Mode

Table 3.1 provides several modes of activities that are potential aerobic exercises. All the suggestions in that list, which is not comprehensive, involve using large muscle groups for a continuous period of time in a rhythmic fashion. The list involves exercises that increase heart rate and breathing frequency. Note the variety in table 3.1. Are you questioning what is best for you? Let's first consider the different general types of activities and then look at your selection process.

ACSM has divided cardiorespiratory endurance activities into three groups (ACSM 2000). Group one includes activities you can easily maintain at a constant intensity and for which the caloric expenditure is similar between individuals. Examples from group one include walking and cycling—especially if using a treadmill or stationary bike. Exercises in this category are good starting points for a fitness program because the intensity is easy to control and they are simple to do.

Table 3.1   List of Aerobic Activities

Group 1*	Group 2**	Group 3***
Walking	Step aerobics	Ballroom dancing
Jogging	Aerobic dance	Country and western dancing
Biking (stationary bike)	Hiking	Tennis
Stair stepping (machine)	Water aerobics	Racquetball
Elliptical training (machine)	Water running	Volleyball
Nordic skiing (machine)	Swimming	Basketball
Running	Cross-country skiing	Soccer

*Group 1: Activities that can be readily maintained at a constant intensity and interindividual variation in energy expenditure is relatively low (ACSM 2000).
**Group 2: Activities in which the rate of energy expenditure is highly relative to skill, but for a given individual can provide a constant intensity (ACSM 2000).
***Group 3: Activities where both skill and intensity of exercise are highly variable (ACSM 2000).

Adapted, by permission, from American College of Sports Medicine (ACSM), 2000, *ACSM's guidelines for exercise testing and prescription, 6th edition* (Baltimore: Lippincott Williams & Wilkins), 144; adapted, by permission, from V.H. Heyward, 2002, *Advanced fitness assessment and exercise prescription, 4th ed.* (Champaign, IL: Human Kinetics), 89.

Group two activities are more skill dependent and include activities in which, with the necessary proficiency, you can maintain a constant intensity. Because of differences in skill levels, the energy expenditure can vary greatly between individuals (ACSM 2000). An example from group two includes swimming because a certain ability level is required to allow a person to maintain the activity for a continuous period of time. Those unskilled in swimming may be able to continue for only very short periods of time before stopping. However, those with sufficient skills can maintain the activity for longer periods of time, allowing swimming to be an excellent endurance exercise. Other activities in this category include cross-country skiing, water aerobics, step aerobics, and hiking.

Group three includes activities with variations in both skill requirements and exercise intensity (ACSM 2000). Examples from group three include tennis, racquetball, dancing, basketball, and other group exercises. The intensity is more difficult to control, especially when competition enters into the picture. Yet, these activities may provide for good variety and do allow for a potential conditioning effect.

Obviously, a wide range of activities potentially allows for improvements in your cardiorespiratory fitness. Having a list is helpful, but you may still be wondering how to decide specifically what you should do. First, ask yourself these two simple questions: "Do I enjoy doing the activity?" and "Do I have access if special equipment or facilities are needed?" One key factor, often overlooked when starting an exercise program, is to find something you enjoy doing and then verify that you have access to the activity. For example, if you have swimming skills, enjoy swimming, but find that the available pool hours do not match your schedule, it will be futile to include swimming in your exercise program. Equally defeating is including stationary cycling, although a potentially wonderful activity for aerobic conditioning, if you cringe at the thought of sitting on a bike for more than 10 minutes and going nowhere. We have observed many exercise programs derail when these two simple questions are not answered affirmatively in the beginning. Choose activities that are both enjoyable and accessible.

The mode of exercise selected should also reflect your current fitness level and health status. If you are just beginning your exercise program, then we recommend you start with group one activities. These activities

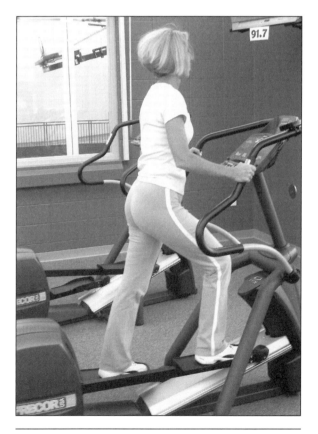

The options are numerous when you're investigating different types of aerobic exercise.

allow you to build a foundation on which you can later move to activities in group two and group three if so desired. Staying with group one activities is also an option, as the groupings do not represent an optimal progression but rather simply different types of activities. For those who already have a cardiorespiratory fitness base, you can continue with group one activities but also may desire to develop skills to allow inclusion of group two or group three options to increase variety in your workout plans.

Determining Appropriate Intensity

Determination of exercise intensity is the next step. This involves consideration of your current health status as well as your overall goals. We discuss the potential need for physician clearance before beginning, as well as how to estimate your current fitness and select the optimal intensity for you.

Obtaining physician clearance. Safety of an exercise program is always a number one priority. With this in mind, ACSM has recommended, in some cases, clearance from a physician before starting. The recommendations are based on your workout goals as well as your current age and risk for heart disease. We will walk you through these recommendations so you will know if you should meet with your physician before starting your exercise program (ACSM 2000).

Determining your workout goals is the first factor to consider. We recommend that most individuals embark on a moderate exercise program. Moderate exercise is defined as activity within your current capacity that can be maintained for 30 to 45 minutes. It involves activity that starts at an easy level and then gradually increases (ACSM 2000). An example of moderate exercise would be a walking program. Some individuals desire, however, to begin a vigorous exercise program such as jogging or running. This is described by ACSM as presenting a "substantial cardiorespiratory challenge," and the need for a physical exam is increased if you want to begin a vigorous program (ACSM 2000).

Understanding your risk for coronary artery disease is another important factor to consider. Table 3.2 includes a list of risk factors for heart disease. Examine the list and check off each risk factor that applies to you. Determine your total risk by subtracting the negative risk factor from the number of positive risk factors.

To determine if a physical exam is necessary before initiation of your exercise program, you must consider your exercise level (moderate or vigorous) and age as well as the number of heart disease risk factors you have. The following are situations in which you would not necessarily need a medical examination before beginning:

- If you are younger than 55 years of age, have zero or one risk factor, and want to start either a moderate or vigorous exercise program

Table 3.2 Heart Disease Risk Factors for Women

Positive risk factors	Definition	Your risk*
Family history	Heart attack, bypass surgery, or sudden cardiac death before the age of 55 in father, brother, or son or before the age of 65 in mother, sister, or daughter	
Cigarette smoking	Current smoker or those who quit within the last 6 months	
High blood pressure[a]	Systolic blood pressure higher than 140 mmHg or diastolic blood pressure higher than 90 mmHg, confirmed on two separate occasions or on blood pressure (antihypertensive) medication	
Dyslipidemia[b]	LDL greater than 130 mg/dL or HDL less than 40 mg/dL or total cholesterol greater than 200 mg/dL or on cholesterol-lowering medication	
Impaired fasting glucose	Fasting glucose (sugar) higher than 100 mg/dL, confirmed on two separate occasions	
Obesity	Body mass index[c] of more than 30 kg/m^2 or waist girth of more than 88 cm (34.6 in.) or waist to hip ratio[d] greater than .86	
Sedentary lifestyle	Anyone not participating in a regular exercise program or who does not meet the Surgeon General's recommendation to accumulate at least 30 min of physical activity on most days of the week	
Negative risk factor	**Definition**	
High HDL cholesterol	HDL cholesterol higher than 60 mg/dL	
TOTAL	Add the number of checks for positive risk factors and then subtract any negative risk factor to get your overall risk.	

*Mark the box with a check if the definition fits your situation.

[a]Blood pressure includes two numbers. The top number is the systolic blood pressure, and it represents the pressure in the blood vessels when the heart is contracting. The bottom number is the diastolic blood pressure, and it represents the pressure in the blood vessels when the heart is between beats. High blood pressure (aka hypertension) can be due to either a high systolic blood pressure or a high diastolic blood pressure, or both.

[b]Cholesterol is recorded with varying degrees of specificity. You may know only your total cholesterol level, and that can be helpful in determining risk (increased risk if total cholesterol is greater than 200 mg/dL). If you have more detailed information about the low-density lipoproteins (LDLs) and the high-density lipoproteins (HDLs), that is even better. LDL cholesterol is the "bad" cholesterol with regard to coronary heart disease. LDL information is preferred over a total cholesterol reading. HDL cholesterol is the "good" cholesterol. If it is low, it is a positive risk factor, and if it is high, it decreases your risk (is a negative risk factor).

cBody mass index (BMI) incorporates both height and weight into a single value expressed in kilograms per meter squared. To determine your BMI, you need to know your current height and weight. If you know these measurements in inches and pounds, you need to convert them to kilograms (kg) and meters (m). To convert pounds to kilograms, simply divide your body weight in pounds by 2.2. To convert inches to meters, multiply your height in inches by .0254. To determine your BMI, take your body weight in kilograms and divide it by the square of your body weight. Follow these steps to calculate your BMI:

      Body weight = _____ pounds

      Height = _____ inches

      Convert body weight in pounds to kg: [# pounds] divided by 2.2 = _____ kg

      Convert height in inches to meters: [# inches] multiplied by .0254 = _____ m

      Square your height in meters: [# meters] $\times$ [# meters] = _____ m^2

            Note: You can also use a calculator with a "square key" (normally shown as x^2).

      Calculate BMI: [weight in kg] divided by [height in m^2] = _____

dThe waist to hip ratio is determined by dividing the circumference of the waist by the circumference of the hips. Use a flexible tape measure to determine the narrowest part of the torso (above the belly button but below the lower part of the breast bone or sternum). Then determine the maximal girth of the hips or buttocks region. Take the measurement for the waist and divide it by the measurement for the hips to determine the waist to hip ratio.

Adapted, by permission, from American College of Sports Medicine (ACSM), 2005, *ACSM's guidelines for exercise texting and prescription, 7th edition* (Baltimore: Lippincott Williams & Wilkins), 15.

- If you are younger than 55 years of age, with two or more risk factors, and want to start a moderate exercise program
- If you are more than 55 years of age, have zero or one risk factor, and plan to start a moderate exercise program

Of course, there is nothing wrong with having a medical examination or a physician's clearance before beginning an exercise program; it simply is not considered a requirement for women in these three categories.

For women over the age of 55 or those younger than 55 with two or more risk factors, physician clearance is recommended before beginning a vigorous exercise program. Also, if you have a known disease (e.g., heart disease, lung disease, diabetes, thyroid disorder, kidney or liver disease), it is recommended that you have a medical examination before starting any exercise program, moderate or vigorous. Realize that these are simply guidelines and that discussing your fitness program with your physician is always encouraged. If you have any questions or special concerns unique to your situation, your physician is a good resource to consult.

Evaluating your current fitness level. Evaluating your current fitness level provides a more precise determination of the most appropriate intensity level for you. Evaluation methods range from precise physician-supervised measurements to simple tests you can conduct yourself to estimate your cardiorespiratory fitness. As described previously, needing a physician clearance before beginning an exercise program depends on your health and fitness status. If physician clearance is not necessary or if clearance has been given, then an evaluation of your current fitness level is the next step.

Laboratory tests, involving breathing through a mouthpiece and analysis of the amount of oxygen you have consumed, allow for precise determination of your cardiorespiratory fitness. Such tests directly measure maximal oxygen consumption ($\dot{V}O_2$max), which is a standard marker of aerobic fitness. $\dot{V}O_2$max is the number of milliliters of oxygen consumed by your body per kilogram of your body weight each minute. The abbreviation for this unit of measurement is ml/kg/min. The more oxygen your body can take in and use during maximal exercise, the higher your $\dot{V}O_2$max reading will be, and the fitter you are. Although highly accurate, actual $\dot{V}O_2$max tests are unnecessary for most women desiring to start an exercise program. In addition, these tests can be rather pricey (likely $200-500) and are typically only available at hospitals and university research labs.

For a more practical analysis of cardiorespiratory fitness, simpler estimations of $\dot{V}O_2$max can be made from nonlaboratory tests, or field tests. These tests can be done on any flat, marked course and include walking or jogging rather than maximal-level exertion. If you have not been performing any physical activity, it is recommended you start a gradually progressive walking program before doing the walking test described in the following paragraphs.

The one-mile walk test requires you to walk one mile on a measured course and then take your pulse at the end of the mile (ACSM 2000). The goal is to walk the mile in the fastest time possible. The time to complete your walk and your postwalk heart rate will be used to estimate your cardiorespiratory fitness. Listed here are the steps to conduct the test. Note that it is easier to do this test with a partner who times your walk and pulse count.

1. Warm up with some slow walking and stretching.
2. Partner will say, "Ready . . . go," then start a stopwatch at the beginning of the course.
3. Complete the one-mile course. You may use a track or any flat, measured course.
4. When you finish the course, the timer will note the time to the nearest second.
5. Immediately after finishing, the timer will ask you to find your pulse (see the sidebar on page 44 for details on taking your pulse). Once you are ready, the timer will say, "Begin," indicating you should start counting your pulse; after 10 seconds the timer will say, "Stop." Record the number of pulses you counted in this 10-second period.

The next step is to calculate your estimated $\dot{V}O_2max$. Please see the sidebar on page 45 for the steps in the calculation. These calculations can be used for women between the ages of 30 and 69 years of age. The higher your $\dot{V}O_2max$, the better your cardiorespiratory fitness. See table 3.3 to see how you compare with other women your age. Do not be discouraged if you are in a lower fitness category—that simply means you have room to improve. If you are already above average, then strive to maintain that edge.

As an example, we have included results for Sally, a 55-year-old post-menopausal woman. Sally's medical history and fitness test results are given in the sidebar on page 53, which includes all the components of designing a cardiorespiratory fitness program, along with the associated calculations, described in this chapter. When we consult table 3.3 for Sally, we see that her $\dot{V}O_2max$ estimate of 29.8 ml/kg/min places her slightly above the 60th percentile for women 50 to 59 years of age. Therefore, Sally is slightly above average in her fitness level.

Table 3.3   Percentile Values for Maximal Aerobic Fitness in Women

Percentile*	Age (years)				
	20-29	30-39	40-49	50-59	60 and above
90	44.2	41.0	39.5	35.2	35.2
80	41.0	38.6	36.3	32.3	31.2
70	38.1	36.7	33.8	30.9	29.4
60	36.7	34.6	32.3	29.4	27.2
50	35.2	33.8	30.9	28.2	25.8
40	33.8	32.3	29.5	26.9	24.5
30	32.3	30.5	28.3	25.5	23.8
20	30.6	28.7	26.5	24.3	22.8
10	28.4	26.5	25.1	22.3	20.8

*The following verbal descriptors are associated with the percentile ranks:
90 = well above average
70 = above average
50 = average
30 = below average
10 = well below average

Adapted, by permission, from American College of Sports Medicine (ACSM), 2000, *ACSM's guidelines for exercise testing and prescription, 6th edition* (Baltimore: Lippincott Williams & Wilkins), 77.

Determining Heart Rate

Finding a pulse. Finding your pulse involves locating a spot where an artery is close to the surface of the skin. The pulse you feel at those locations corresponds with the beating of your heart. We have listed a couple of locations where the pulse is easiest to find.

Radial Artery Pulse

▸ Rotate your hands so palms are facing up.

▸ Take your left hand and wrap it around the wrist of your right arm (keep both palms up).

▸ Place the fingers of your left hand on the thumb side of your right wrist. (Note: There is a slight groove between some tendons in the middle of the wrist and the radius bone, which leads toward your thumb—your fingers should be in that groove.)

▸ Squeeze slightly with your left hand; you should feel your radial pulse.

Carotid Artery Pulse

▸ Place the fingers of your right hand on the center of your neck on your windpipe.

▸ Slide your fingers to one side of your neck until you feel the pulse of your carotid artery (about an inch or so off center).

▸ Use only very light pressure when taking a carotid pulse because pushing too hard can make it difficult to feel the pulse and also can potentially change your heart rhythm.

▸ Also, take a pulse on only one side at a time because the blood flowing through the carotid arteries nourishes your brain; you do not want to limit blood flow through both carotid arteries at the same time.

Select one of these locations to find your pulse. Count the number of pulses for 10 seconds. This number of pulses needs to be multiplied by 6 to determine a total number of beats for one minute (because 10 seconds × 6 will give us a total for 60 seconds, which is one minute).

Heart rate monitors. With today's technical advances, heart rate can also be determined with a simple device (a special strap worn around the torso just under the breasts). The electrical activity associated with each heartbeat is picked up by this device and transmitted to a receiver that looks like a watch. The number displayed on the receiver is your heart rate in units of beats per minute (so there is no need to multiply by 6 as you did when taking your pulse manually for 10 seconds). Heart rate monitor prices have dropped considerably since they first appeared on the exercise scene. Simple models can be purchased for approximately $30 to $40. Using a heart rate monitor allows for continuous readings; this is an advantage over manually taking your pulse.

Calculating V̇O₂max From the One-Mile Walk Test for Women

Information needed:

Body weight in pounds = _____

Age in years = _____

Mile time in minutes* = _____

Heart rate in beats per minute = _____

*You will have originally recorded time in minutes and seconds but will need to insert your time here in minutes (with seconds shown as decimal numbers—in other words, a particular fraction of a minute). To do this, insert the number of seconds beyond the last minute mark recorded into this formula:

[# seconds] × **100** = _____ divided by **60** = _____ divided by **100** = # of seconds as a decimal

Insert your recorded information into each line.

[body weight in pounds] × **.0769** =   _____

[age in years] × **.3877** =   _____

[mile time in minutes] × **3.2649** =   _____

[heart rate in beats per minute] × **.1565** =   _____

TOTAL = _____

132.853 – [TOTAL] = your V̇O₂max estimation

Note: All numbers in bold print are constants and are predetermined values for the calculations.

Calculating exercise intensity. Once you know your estimated V̇O₂max, you can determine what intensity will be appropriate for your fitness level. The typical recommendation is to exercise in a range of 50 to 85 percent of your V̇O₂max (ACSM 2000). This range will be unique to you and should be determined from the results of your one-mile walk test. Take your estimated V̇O₂max and multiply it by .50 and .85 to determine your specific range. See the sidebar on page 46 for a guide to calculating your exercise intensity range. In our example (see Sally's Example, page 53), Sally's V̇O₂max was estimated to be 29.8 ml/kg/min, so the target range for Sally would be 14.9 to 25.3 ml/kg/min.

Selecting Your Exercise Intensity

The typical recommendation for exercise intensity is 50 to 85 percent of your $\dot{V}O_2$max. Fill in the blanks to determine your range based on the results from your one-mile walk:

$\dot{V}O_2$max estimation = _____ ml/kg/min (take this from the final calculation in the sidebar on calculating $\dot{V}O_2$max from the one-mile walk test)

[$\dot{V}O_2$max estimate] $\times$ .50 = _____ ml/kg/min (low end of intensity range)

[$\dot{V}O_2$max estimate] $\times$ .85 = _____ ml/kg/min (high end of intensity range)

Now you will convert the ml/kg/min to METs (metabolic equivalents, a simpler unit that will allow you to tailor your exercise intensity more easily) for both the low and high end of your intensity range:

[Low end $\dot{V}O_2$] divided by **3.5** = _____ METs (low end of intensity range)

[High end $\dot{V}O_2$] divided by **3.5** = _____ METs (high end of intensity range)

These values can be used to select your activity level from table 3.4. Start at the lower end of your intensity range, and gradually move toward activity at the higher end of the range.

$\dot{V}O_2$max is expressed in milliliters of oxygen per kilogram of body weight per minute. To easily determine the intensity level of particular activities, one more calculation is required. Take the $\dot{V}O_2$max value you calculated and divide it by 3.5. This changes the units from ml/kg/min to METs. See the sidebar on this page to convert your $\dot{V}O_2$max estimate into METs. One MET equals the oxygen requirement of the body at rest. This conversion to METs translates your $\dot{V}O_2$max into an easier unit—simply a multiple of your body's oxygen use at rest. MET values for various activities are available in many published tables (see list in the resources section at the end of the book). For selected activities, see table 3.4. In our example, Sally would want to exercise between 4 and 7 METs (see full explanation of this determination in Sally's Example, page 53) and thus could select walking on a treadmill at 4.5 miles per hour, allowing her to train at an intensity level within the recommended range. One more benefit of knowing the MET value for activities is your ability to estimate the number of calories you are burning during the activity (ACSM 2000). We discuss how to determine this, as well as how to use this information to modify or individualize your exercise program, later in the chapter.

Table 3.4 MET Levels for Selected Activities

Activity	METs used
Bicycling outdoors, <10.0 mph, leisure riding	4.0
Bicycling outdoors, 10.0-11.9 mph	6.0
Bicycling outdoors, 12.0-13.9 mph	8.0
Bicycling outdoors, 14.0-15.9 mph	10.0
Biking, stationary, 50 watts, very light effort	3.0
Biking, stationary, 100 watts, light effort	5.5
Biking, stationary, 150 watts, moderate effort	7.0
Biking, stationary, 200 watts, vigorous effort	10.5
Running, 5 mph	8.0
Running, 6 mph	10.0
Running, 7 mph	11.5
Running, 8 mph	13.5
Swimming laps, freestyle, moderate to light effort	8.0
Swimming laps, sidestroke	8.0
Swimming laps, backstroke	8.0
Swimming laps, breaststroke	10.0
Swimming laps, butterfly	11.0
Walking, 2.0 mph	2.5
Walking, 2.5 mph	3.0
Walking, 3.0 mph	3.5
Walking, 3.5 mph	4.0
Walking, 4.5 mph	4.5

Adapted, by permission, from American College of Sports Medicine (ACSM), 2000, *ACSM's guidelines for exercise testing and prescription, 4th edition* (Baltimore: Lippincott Williams & Wilkins), 674-681.

In addition to using MET values to determine intensity, other measures can also assist with adjusting your exercise load. Differences in environmental temperature or your level of hydration may influence your body's response to a particular activity, so considering heart rate and rating of perceived exertion becomes important (ACSM 2000). We discuss each of these measures now in more detail.

Heart rate is simply the number of times the heart beats in a minute (see sidebar on page 44 for information on how to measure your heart rate). Heart rate is a very useful indicator of intensity, and we typically prescribe target exercise heart rates within a range of 70 to 85 percent of maximal heart rate. You likely do not have an actual measured maximal heart rate and thus will need to estimate it. Subtracting your age from 220 is one way to get an estimate. See the sidebar on page 49 for steps to calculate your maximal heart rate and your heart rate range. For Sally, who is 55 years of age, her predicted maximal heart rate is 165 beats per minute (220 − 55 = 165). So, Sally would start with a target heart rate range of 115 to 140 beats per minute (see sidebar on page 53 for a full description). Since this is an age prediction rather than an actual measurement, the potential for some variability exists (10-15 beats in either direction), but do not discount the benefit of monitoring your heart rate because it does give you a good indication of your exertion level. Realize that this calculation will also be altered if you are taking certain medications (e.g., beta blockers taken for high blood pressure or other conditions will result in a lower heart rate than would be expected for your age). The calculated range serves as a guideline in conjunction with the rating of perceived exertion.

Rating of perceived exertion (RPE) is a numerical ranking used to subjectively rate your feelings during exercise. It is your bodywide feeling of exertion and can be helpful in guiding exercise intensity. RPE is useful when it is difficult to measure heart rate or when a person is on a medication that influences heart rate. (For example, a heart medication called a beta blocker depresses heart rate, while caffeine elevates heart rate.) The RPE scale is shown in figure 3.2. The recommended RPE associated with sufficient intensity for a cardiorespiratory benefit is

6	No exertion at all
7	
8	Extremely light
9	Very light
10	
11	Light
12	
13	Somewhat hard
14	
15	Hard (heavy)
16	
17	Very hard
18	
19	Extremely hard
20	Maximal exertion

Borg RPE scale
© Gunnar Borg, 1970, 1985, 1994, 1998

Figure 3.2   Borg's rating of perceived exertion scale.

G. Borg, 1998, *Borg's perceived exertion and pain scales* (Champaign, IL: Human Kinetics), 47.

12 to 16 (ACSM 2000). The verbal descriptors for this range include "somewhat hard" to "hard."

The use of MET charts, heart rate ranges, and RPE can help you select and maintain appropriate exercise intensity. The MET charts are a good place for you to start. You then can adjust the workload based on your heart rate responses and your subjective feelings as represented by RPE. Another very simple way to consider intensity is the talk test. This simply means that as you exercise, you should be able to talk with someone. If you are gasping for breath after every word or two, your intensity is definitely too high. If you can recite the Gettysburg Address without a break or hesitation, your intensity may not be sufficient (although your memory is wonderful).

Determining Your Heart Rate Range

You probably do not have a direct measurement of your maximal heart rate, so you will estimate your maximal heart rate by subtracting your age from 220.

220 − [your age] = _____ beats per minute = HRmax

For cardiorespiratory fitness, the target heart rate range prescription during exercise is between 70 and 85 percent of maximum. Calculate your range as follows:

[Your estimated HRmax] × .70 = _____ (low end of heart rate range)

[Your estimated HRmax] × .85 = _____ (high end of heart rate range)

As you exercise, keep your heart rate within this range. Use your heart rate range in conjunction with subjective feelings of the exercise (RPE scale; see figure 3.2). For RPE, focus on maintaining your workload from levels 12 to 16.

Targeting a Reasonable Duration

The duration of the endurance phase of your workout will be determined by practical aspects such as how much time you have to exercise as well as your current level of fitness and the intensity level with which you are most comfortable. The interrelationship between duration and intensity is inverse. That means with long duration, the intensity will be lower, but for short duration, the intensity may be higher. The minimum intensity for cardiorespiratory benefits appears to be approximately 50 percent of $\dot{V}O_2$max or even slightly below that for those who have been completely inactive, or sedentary.

For beginners, the initial goal is not about intensity or exact time but rather to develop baseline fitness. If you are just beginning an exercise program, focus on selecting an activity at an intensity you can maintain for 10 to 15 minutes. Do not start with an arbitrary goal of 30 or 45 minutes;

just focus on 10 to 15 minutes. You can even break that into three 5-minute periods, including a rest between. As that becomes easier, add a few minutes per workout session. Continue adding a few minutes until you are easily completing 30 minutes of exercise per session. At this point you can either continue to add time or you can consider increasing the intensity slightly. We have included a diagram that will be helpful in your progression from beginner to established exerciser (see figure 3.3).

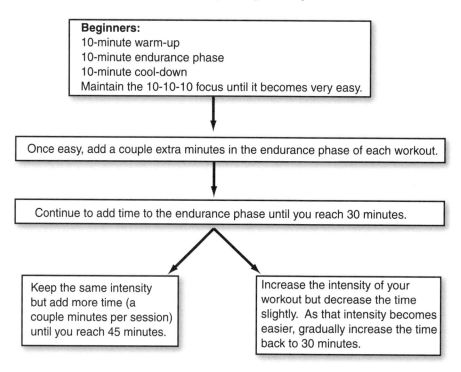

Figure 3.3 Exercise flow from beginner to established exerciser.

For those who have already established a baseline level of fitness, you should focus on completing 20 to 60 minutes of aerobic activity. If you are exercising for a shorter duration, near the 20-minute end of the range, consider maintaining your intensity at the higher end of your calculated range. Always compare your intensity with RPE to ensure the workload is not too difficult. For those who are more comfortable with or prefer the lower end of the intensity range, consider a longer duration such as 45 minutes for the endurance phase of your workout.

Finding an Effective Frequency

How often you perform aerobic activity is termed the frequency. So far you have selected a mode of exercise you enjoy and can conveniently access, and you've determined the right balance of intensity and time per exercise session. Now you must consider how many days per week you will complete your aerobic exercise training. Gains in fitness appear to increase as the frequency of exercise increases. Should you exercise seven days per week for the best return? Most likely, the answer is no. The amount of improvement in cardiorespiratory fitness starts to plateau beyond three days per week, and at the same time, the risk of orthopedic problems may start to increase (ACSM 1998b). Therefore, the concept of a "work-a-day-then-rest-a day" routine (Howley and Franks 2003) is suggested. ACSM recommendations include three to five workouts per week (ACSM 2000). Realize if you have other goals (e.g., weight loss or competitive sports) the frequency may be increased.

Creating Your Exercise Plan

The combination of mode, intensity, duration, and frequency is your aerobic exercise prescription. The selection of each component allows you to determine the calories used during the activity. Calories used (also referred to as caloric expenditure) is a more global view of your workout, allowing for a type of workout summary. The ACSM recommends a target range of 150 to 400 calories be expended in physical activity per day (ACSM 2000). As a beginner, you would target the lower end of the range. Once at a higher fitness level, your goal would be the upper end of the range, 300 to 400 calories per day.

Caloric expenditure is influenced by some factors that cannot be directly measured, including your skill level and coordination. For example, as a beginning jogger you will likely be less efficient than an experienced runner. Thus the calories expended to jog at the same speed would be more for the beginner compared with the experienced athlete who has learned over time to focus all muscle activity toward the act of jogging. The inability to measure this will limit how precise the estimation will be. The following equation allows you to approximate how many calories your activity will cost you per minute (see sidebar on page 52 for steps in calculating your own caloric expenditure).

$$(\text{METs} \times \textbf{3.5} \times \text{body weight in kilograms})/\textbf{200} = \text{calories per minute}$$

For example, if Sally walks on the treadmill at 4.5 miles per hour for 35 minutes, she will expend almost 200 calories (see Sally's Example for how Sally calculated this). If Sally wants to expend about the same number of calories but would rather walk slower, she could also walk at 3.5 miles per hour but would need to walk for slightly more than 40 minutes rather than 35 minutes. By using the information in a MET table (such as that found in table 3.4), you can estimate the calories burned during your workout. This not only can be useful from a nutritional perspective but also allows an overall view of the workout because caloric use reflects both the time and intensity of a particular exercise mode.

Calculating Calorie Costs of an Activity

You must know the MET level of the activity and your body weight in kilograms.

[METs for your activity] $\times$ **3.5** $\times$ [body weight in kilograms] = _____
divided by **200** = _____ kcal/min

Note: kcal/min is the estimated number of calories you will have burned each minute of your activity. To determine the total calories burned for your workout, multiply this number by the number of minutes you did the activity.

[# kcal/min] $\times$ [# minutes of the activity] = _____ kcal burned in the workout

Cool-Down

We have discussed the warm-up as the appetizer, the endurance phase as the main course, and now the cool-down will be likened to a healthy dessert. The cool-down is the finishing touch to a great workout. Our dessert analogy may crumble here because every workout should include a cool-down (unfortunately, not every dessert is healthy, and not every meal includes a dessert). Activities included in a cool-down are similar to those of the warm-up; however, the intensity throughout the cool-down should gradually diminish. As with the warm-up, there are a number of physiological benefits for a cool-down, including the following (ACSM 2000):

- Allows for the heart to slow down in a controlled manner, helping to avoid negative changes in the heart rhythm
- Prevents drops in blood pressure, which can occur when activity is stopped abruptly
- Helps to gradually decrease body temperature, which will have naturally increased during the endurance phase

This list clearly shows the practical issues (i.e., you don't want to faint if your blood pressure drops) as well as safety issues (i.e., avoiding negative alterations in your heart rhythm) that a proper cool-down will address.

Cool-down activities are similar to those in the warm-up and include low-intensity aerobic exercise, calisthenics, and stretching. The key with selecting your cool-down components is to gradually decrease the intensity. The cool-down is the "off-ramp" of the workout and should slowly return your body, as observed with breathing frequency and heart rate, to preexercise levels. For example, including walking after a jogging workout will allow your breathing frequency to slow down and your heart rate to move toward preexercise levels. Following a decrease in your heart rate and breathing, stretching activities are also very appropriate and should include the arms and shoulders, torso (upper and lower), neck, and hips (ACSM 2000). (See chapter 5 for specific suggestions on total body stretches.)

Sally's Example

BACKGROUND

Sally is a 55-year-old, 2 years postmenopause. She is somewhat active in her job as an elementary teacher. She wants to start a moderate-intensity exercise program. She weighs 150 pounds and is five feet, eight inches tall.

BMI CALCULATION

Sally's BMI is 22.8 and is calculated below (BMI = kg/m^2):

Body weight = 150 pounds = 68.18 kg (note: pounds divided by 2.2 gives kg)

Height = 68 inches = 1.73 meters (note: inches multiplied by .0254 gives meters)

Square the height: 1.73 $\times$ 1.73 = 2.99

BMI = 68.18 divided by 2.99 = 22.8 kg/m^2

RISK FACTOR ASSESSMENT

Sally's father had bypass surgery at the age of 54. She has never smoked cigarettes; she has a total cholesterol of 190 mg/dl, an HDL of 65, and a resting blood pressure of 124/78. When considering Sally's risk level for heart disease, she has one positive risk factor (family history) and one negative risk factor (high HDL), so her risk factor total is zero. Thus, Sally can begin either a moderate or vigorous exercise program without the necessity of a physical examination before beginning.

ONE-MILE FITNESS TEST

Sally completes a one-mile course at her school in 15 minutes and 45 seconds. To convert her time from seconds to tenths of a minute, she would need to insert the 45 seconds in the following calculation (numbers in bold are the constants):

45 $\times$ **100** = 4,500 divided by **60** = 75 divided by **100** = .75

Thus for Sally, her mile time in minutes would be 15.75.

(continued)

(continued)

Sally's 10-second pulse count at the end of the one-mile walk is 20. She multiplies 20 × 6 to determine her heart rate in beats per minute to be 120. Her calculations for $\dot{V}O_2$max follow:

[body weight in pounds is 150] ×**.0769** =   11.5350
[age in years is 55] × **.3877** =   21.3235
[time in minutes is 15.75] × **3.2649** =   51.4222
[heart rate in beats per minute is 120] × **.1565** = 18.7800

TOTAL = 103.0607

132.853 − 103.0607 = 29.8 = $\dot{V}O_2$max estimation

To calculate the target range, Sally takes her estimated $\dot{V}O_2$max of 29.3 ml/kg/min and multiplies it by .50 (for the lower end of her target range at 50 percent) and .85 (for the upper end of her target range at 85 percent).

50% $\dot{V}O_2$max for Sally = 29.8 × .50 = 14.9 ml/kg/min

85% $\dot{V}O_2$max for Sally = 29.8 × .85 = 25.3 ml/kg/min

MET DETERMINATION

To calculate METs, so she can use table 3.4 to pick out activities, Sally converts the $\dot{V}O_2$max values from ml/kg/min to METs by dividing each value by 3.5 as follows:

14.9 ml/kg/min divided by **3.5** = 4.3 METs

25.3 ml/kg/min divided by **3.5** = 7.2 METs

This gives Sally a target zone range of 4.3 to 7.2 METs. Sally decides to start with treadmill walking and selects 4.5 miles per hour, which is equal to 4.5 METs (see table 3.4 on page 47).

CALORIC EXPENDITURE ESTIMATION

To calculate the number of calories she will burn by walking 4.5 miles per hour for 35 minutes, Sally uses the following formula:

(METs × **3.5** × body weight in kilograms)/**200** = calories per minute

First she will convert her weight in pounds (150) to kilograms. This is done by taking her weight in pounds and dividing by 2.2. Thus her weight in kilograms is 68.18. She now can use the previous formula to calculate the number of calories burned per minute.

For Sally, (4.5 METs × **3.5** × 68.18 kg)/**200** = 5.4 calories per minute. If Sally exercises for 35 minutes, she simply multiplies the total time by the calories burned per minute as follows:

5.4 calories per minute × 35 minutes = 189 calories

INTENSITY CHECKS: HEART RATE AND RPE

Sally is 55 years old and does not have a direct measurement of her maximal heart rate, so she will be estimating this by subtracting her age from 220.

$$220 - 55 = 165 \text{ beats per minute}$$

Sally's estimated maximal heart rate is 165. For cardiorespiratory fitness, the target heart rate range prescription during exercise is between 70 and 85 percent of maximum. Sally calculates her target heart rate range as follows:

$$165 \times .70 = 115$$

$$165 \times .85 = 140$$

As Sally exercises, she wants to maintain her heart rate between 115 and 140 beats per minute. This guides her exercise in conjunction with her subjective feelings of the exercise, which she quantifies using the RPE scale (see figure 3.2 on page 48). She focuses on maintaining her workload between RPE levels 12 and 16.

FINE-TUNING THE WORKOUT

Sally uses her heart rate and RPE to fine-tune this workout selection. She finds that both her heart rate (138 beats per minute) and her RPE (15) are on the higher end of the recommended ranges. She also finds that walking at 4.5 miles per hour is a bit fast for her to enjoy. Sally could decrease the speed to a more comfortable pace and try a small grade (incline) on the treadmill until her RPE and heart rate lower a bit. To still get the same overall benefit, she could also reduce the intensity (represented by the speed of the treadmill) and increase the total time. If she selects 3.5 miles per hour as a comfortable treadmill pace, let's determine the number of minutes she will need to walk. First she needs to see how 3.5 miles per hour is related to METs. Using table 3.4, she sees that 3.5 miles per hour is 4.0 METs. Once again Sally plugs the numbers into the equation:

$$(4.0 \text{ METs} \times \textbf{3.5} \times 68.18 \text{ kg})/\textbf{200} = 4.8 \text{ calories per minute}$$

To expend at least 200 calories at this pace, Sally needs to exercise for just over 40 minutes (**200** calories divided by 4.8 calories per minute = 42 minutes).

Summary

Aerobic exercise is beneficial from an overall health standpoint and in particular has many benefits for women, especially during menopause. Your program should be individualized to your health status and your fitness goals. If you have not been active previously, the opportunity for cardiorespiratory fitness gains is very real. Periodically repeating the one-mile walk test is recommended to allow you to update your status. Chapters 6 and 8 include more detailed discussion on specific activities and tracking your progress.

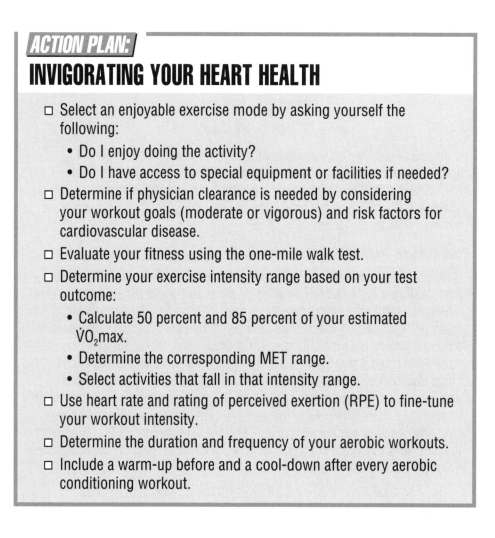

ACTION PLAN:
INVIGORATING YOUR HEART HEALTH

☐ Select an enjoyable exercise mode by asking yourself the following:
  • Do I enjoy doing the activity?
  • Do I have access to special equipment or facilities if needed?
☐ Determine if physician clearance is needed by considering your workout goals (moderate or vigorous) and risk factors for cardiovascular disease.
☐ Evaluate your fitness using the one-mile walk test.
☐ Determine your exercise intensity range based on your test outcome:
  • Calculate 50 percent and 85 percent of your estimated $\dot{V}O_2max$.
  • Determine the corresponding MET range.
  • Select activities that fall in that intensity range.
☐ Use heart rate and rating of perceived exertion (RPE) to fine-tune your workout intensity.
☐ Determine the duration and frequency of your aerobic workouts.
☐ Include a warm-up before and a cool-down after every aerobic conditioning workout.

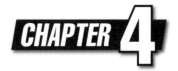

STRENGTHENING POWERFUL WOMEN

Many menopausal women or those approaching menopause do not rank muscular training high on their list of health priorities. You are more likely to be concerned about weight gain, increasing cholesterol, mammograms, hot flashes, and decreased metabolism. In this chapter, we discuss why muscular fitness is increasingly important to women's health before, during, and after menopause.

After reading chapter 3, "Invigorating Your Heart Health," you're well acquainted with the important link between cardiorespiratory fitness and a woman's health and well-being. Muscular fitness, another component of personal fitness and your overall health, includes muscular strength and muscular endurance. Muscular strength is the maximum amount of force that can be produced by a muscle or group of muscles. Muscular endurance is the ability of a muscle or group of muscles to exert force repeatedly over a given time or to maintain a contraction for a period of time. Active people of all ages need both strength and muscular endurance to accomplish tasks of daily living and work requirements, as well as family activities and recreation.

Strength training involves using your muscles against progressively increasing weight over time. You work your muscles when you lift, push, and pull. Muscular fitness is developed as you progressively overload or demand more from your muscles. The practice of overloading the muscles is known by a variety of synonymous names that are used in this chapter: strength training, strength conditioning, weight training, resistance training, and progressive resistance training. Resistance training can include the use of a wide variety of equipment and is limited only by your fitness goals. Free weights (dumbbells, barbells, cans of soup, or plastic gallon jugs filled with water) and isokinetic (specialized equipment found in re-hab centers controlling the speed of movement), isotonic (weightlifting machines, doing push-ups), and isometric (static) training are all used to develop muscular fitness.

Exercises to increase strength are performed by contracting the muscles against an external resistance. Isometric, or static, contraction of the muscles occurs when the muscles are contracted against an immovable object and no movement occurs. For example, if you push against a brick wall, your muscles tighten, but the wall stays in place. When a joint moves and the muscles push, pull, or lift an object through space, dynamic (iso-tonic) muscle contraction occurs. Concentric contraction of the muscles takes place when the muscles shorten to move or lift an object, whereas controlled lowering of the object causes an eccentric contraction when the muscles lengthen. Usually, dynamic muscle contraction is preferred over static because these contractions are used during activities of daily living, and they can help maintain strength throughout the range of mo-tion of the given joint (Singh 2000).

A progressive resistance training (PRT) program places increasingly greater demands on the skeletal muscles. It is this unaccustomed weight that causes the muscles to adapt and become stronger (Singh 2000). A fairly heavy load is used for the strength exercises performed during a well-designed PRT program (Singh 2000).

Benefits of Strength Training

About 40 percent of the body consists of muscles that are used for move-ment, work, and play (Fahey, Insel, and Roth 2003). When your muscles are strong, you can confidently lift, reach, move, push, and pull without much thought. Strong muscles reduce the possibility of injuries, improve body composition, provide a sense of confidence, and allow you to recover more quickly from physical activities (ACSM 2001). In this section, we discuss a number of important reasons for strength training.

Sarcopenia (a reduction in muscle strength and size) occurs as a result of aging. Muscle loss can result from a variety of factors, including inad-equate dietary protein intake, reduced muscular activity, physical inac-tivity, injury, or illness. Middle-aged and older women need to consume adequate amounts of protein to maintain their muscle mass. (For more nutrition information, see chapter 7.)

Weight training programs for women are effective in preserving muscle mass and preventing sarcopenia and the decline of metabolic rate (ACSM 2001). Most health and fitness experts believe that people are never too old to start a resistance training program and will benefit both physically and psychologically from it. And, following the advice of one expert, you are "probably too old *not* to exercise" (Westcott and Baechle 1998, 2).

Most adults will lose between five and seven pounds of muscle every decade (Westcott and Baechle 1998). After women reach the age of 30, decreases in muscle density and increases in intramuscular fat are found in cross-sectional areas of the thighs (ACSM 1998c). This trend continues as lean body mass decreases by approximately 15 percent between the ages of 30 and 80 (Cohn et al. 1980). In general, there is almost a 30 percent decrease in overall strength between the age of 50 and 70 years, with dramatic losses after age 70 (ACSM 1998c). To emphasize this point, research from the Framingham Study shows that 40 percent of women 55 to 64 years old, 45 percent of women in the 65 to 74 age category, and 65 percent of women between the ages of 75 and 84 could not lift 10 pounds (Jette and Branch 1981). Over the years, the result is less functional ability and a higher percentage of body fat, which contribute to a declining metabolic rate.

The good news is that following a well-planned resistance training program increases muscle fiber size in older women (Fleck and Kraemer 1997). Increasing the size of muscle fibers helps combat the age-related sarcopenia that normally occurs in women. Therefore, your resistance training program helps slow this process.

Every decade as you lose muscle tissue, your metabolism also decreases by about 5 percent (Westcott and Baechle 1998). This slower metabolic rate contributes to middle-aged weight gain when you eat the same amount of calories but don't burn all the calories consumed. Strength training can slow the metabolic decreases, muscle loss, and weight gain that normally occur in middle-aged women. Muscle is metabolically active tissue that requires energy (calories). Each day, your body uses more than 35 calories to maintain each pound of muscle, while only 2 calories are needed to sustain a pound of fat (Westcott and Baechle 1998). Therefore, an ongoing resistance training program makes sense so you can maintain or increase your muscle mass and not feel as if you are constantly dieting to maintain a healthy weight as you age. Additionally, no cosmetic surgery, supplements, or special foods are necessary for this achievement.

There's more good news about the benefits of resistance training, especially for women before and after menopause. Strength training is linked to high bone mineral density in adults of all ages and both sexes (ACSM 2004). Osteoporosis is a type of skeletal deterioration, characterized by decreasing bone density that weakens the bone structure (Graves and Franklin 2001). Osteoporosis is partially preventable with adequate amounts of calcium in the diet, along with progressive high-intensity resistance training (Graves and Franklin 2001). Dense, healthy bones are created in a constant rebuilding process as osteoclasts, cells that break down bone, are replaced by osteoblasts, cells that form bone (Graves and Franklin 2001). One way to stimulate the osteoblasts is to repeatedly use greater-than-normal loads on the bones. The amount of bone building is relative to the amount of overload on the bone, so within limits, increases in the overload will cause greater amounts of bone to be formed (Ebben and Jensen 1998, ACSM 2004). New formation of bone develops on the bone's outer surface, creating stronger bones that are less likely to fracture (Graves and Franklin 2001). Incremental bone formation occurs within 8 to 12 weeks of strength training, but four to six months of progressive resistance training is the minimum amount of time needed to increase bone mineral density (Graves and Franklin 2001). The greatest increases in bone density occur in previously inactive postmenopausal women who participate in resistance training (Kerr et al. 2001).

A progressive resistance program can be used for the prevention of osteoporosis or when combined with other osteoporosis treatment programs for postmenopausal women (Kerr et al. 2001). It may help to "achieve the highest possible peak bone mass in premenopausal women, and in maintaining or increasing bone in postmenopausal women" (Singh 2000, 380). According to a variety of research studies, the load (i.e., the amount of resistance placed on the bone and muscles) is more important for improving bone density than the type of exercises (free weights, machines, elastic bands) used in progressive resistance training (Singh 2000). "Improvements in bone density have been seen after training regimens of 1, 2, or 3 days per week, provided the intensity (relative load) is high" (Singh 2000, 381). Because bone loss, muscle loss, and decreases in strength and endurance occur when strength training ends, postmenopausal women are urged to continue regular progressive resistance training as long as their health allows (Singh 2000; ACSM 2004).

Strength training provides still more health benefits (Westcott and Baechle 1998):

- Reduced risk of adult-onset diabetes
- Lower blood pressure
- Decreased arthritis pain
- Maintenance of or improvement in lower back health

Glucose metabolism improves because resistance training contributes to an increased metabolism and the resulting increases in energy needed for larger muscles. After participation in a strength training program, decreases in blood pressure in middle-aged participants have been noted (Westcott and Baechle 1998). Resistance training strengthens the muscles around joints, which aids in joint functioning. These stronger muscles can then absorb and cushion the impact of shock to the joints.

Other clinical outcomes of high-intensity resistance training include the following (Singh 2000):

- Increased functional independence
- Improved gait velocity
- Improved sleep
- Decreased depressive symptoms
- Increased self-efficacy
- Increased overall physical activity level
- Improved static and dynamic balance

In adults there is a strong correlation between desired walking speed and muscular strength (Bassey, Bendall, and Pearson 1988), so resistance training is an effective way to maintain physical activity. Strength conditioning exercises that utilize standing positions while using free weights can increase balance and coordination (ACSM 1998c). Thanks to these types of physiological changes, the postmenopausal woman who was fearful of falls or a broken hip is more likely to believe she can be active without injury (Singh 2000).

In summary, muscle loss reduces your ability to function normally and can become a vicious cycle of decreasing activity and additional muscle loss. To break this cycle, we advise women to use strength conditioning routines that include increasingly heavier weights over time.

Misconceptions About Women and Strength Training

One of the primary misconceptions is that women who lift weights will "bulk up" and look masculine. These fears are unfounded. The reason men can build more muscle mass is because of testosterone. The level of testosterone in women is less than that in men, so equal hypertrophy (muscle growth) will not occur. Additionally, since resistance training increases lean body mass and decreases body fat, there should be no increase in a woman's overall size. Your body weight may remain the same, but you are most likely to notice a difference in the way your clothing fits your leaner, stronger body.

Another mistaken belief that often accompanies a weight training program is "no pain, no gain." This mentality can cause an injury or make an injury worse. No one should lift weights when there is pain in the muscle or joint. Working the muscles will create warmth and a slight burning sensation, but it should not be painful.

A third commonly held myth is that men and women should have different resistance training programs. Male and female bodies have the same muscles—all of which need to be strengthened and developed. The overall goal of the program is to increase, maintain, or regain strength, muscle, and bone density. Healthy women should participate in high-intensity or high-load progressive resistance training. If you lift only light weights, the needed bone building and adaptations in soft tissue (muscle, cartilage, tendons, and ligaments) will not take place (Ebben and Jensen 1998). Focusing on weak areas is important for both men and women. Typically, women have significantly less upper body strength, so more emphasis should be directed at developing these muscle groups.

Another myth of resistance training is that of losing flexibility. When individuals participate in well-designed fitness programs that include cardiorespiratory conditioning, strength training, and stretching exercises, becoming inflexible will not happen. Flexibility in both men and women is either maintained or improved as a result of resistance training programs (Fleck and Kraemer 1997).

Some women believe that good resistance training cannot be completed without a long workout. You can achieve the benefits of a well-designed weight training program in workouts taking less than 30 minutes two or three times a week (Westcott and Baechle 1998). The intensity of the exercise is more important than duration or length of the exercises (Westcott and Baechle 1998).

Because women who participate in strength training activities generally maintain a higher percentage of lean body mass and lower proportion of body fat, self-esteem is generally enhanced. What woman cannot benefit from looking feminine, confident, and strong? There are very few disadvantages to participating in progressive training, so let's find out more about developing a well-designed program.

Principles of Strength Training

In any discussion of muscular strength and endurance, several key terms must be mentioned. These include reversibility, specificity, overload, and intensity. Simply stated, reversibility means "use it or lose it." Muscles atrophy when they are unused and hypertrophy when used for strength and endurance. The principle of specificity refers to the effect of strength training on specific muscles of the body. Weightlifting exercises for your legs will not improve the strength of your arms or upper body. Therefore, 8 to 10 different resistance exercises for the major muscle groups need to be incorporated into your strength training routine. Successful weight training uses the overload principle to progressively increase the resistance placed on the muscles as they become capable of lifting heavier weight (Graves and Franklin 2001).

Your weight training program will consist of repetitions and sets. When you pick up a weight to exercise a muscle, lifting that weight one time is a repetition, or "rep." Lifting the weight multiple times in succession is a set of repetitions, or more commonly called a set. ACSM recommends at least two strength conditioning sessions per week that include a minimum of one set of 8 to 10 repetitions of 8 to 10 different exercises that target the major muscle groups (ACSM 2001).

Intensity in strength training can best be accomplished by progressively increasing the weight or resistance to increase the exertion. More repetitions or more sets don't create a better workout. Most strength gains are made through increasing the resistance. To progress on any strength exercise, you would add a 2 to 10 percent weight increase when you can lift the current weight more than the normal 8 to 12 reps on two consecutive training sessions (ACSM 2002). Then, begin working to increase the number of reps back up to 8 to 12 again.

Medical Concerns and Safety Issues

Now that you know the benefits of an intensive PRT program, let's consider the medical concerns and safety factors. Your present health will dictate whether or not you need to receive medical approval before initiating a strength training program. Certain preexisting health conditions will preclude your participation in a PRT program or may require modifications in your program.

Obtaining Physician Clearance

As recommended in chapter 3, you should consider your current exercise level and possible risk factors in determining whether or not you need a physician's clearance to begin an exercise program. If any of the following health conditions apply, you should receive your physician's approval before beginning a progressive resistance workout (Baechle and Earle 1995, 24):

- Over age 50 and not previously active
- History of heart disease or taking medication for heart conditions
- High blood pressure or taking blood pressure medication
- History of respiratory problems or asthma
- Surgery or bone, muscle, tendon, or ligament problems that would be aggravated by weight training

Of course, even if none of these conditions exist, inform your physician of your training at your next annual physical exam.

Contraindications to Progressive Resistance Training

Overall, resistance training is a safe form of exercise, and almost everyone from adolescents to the elderly should include it in their fitness programs. Unless there is a medical reason not to participate, people with low levels of initial strength will benefit from resistance training. Medical contraindications to progressive resistance training include the following conditions (Singh 2000, 50):

- Angina (chest pain), low blood pressure, or arrhythmias (abnormal heart rhythms) caused by resistance training
- Severe valvular heart disease
- Cerebral aneurysm
- Recent intracerebral or subdural hemorrhage
- Uncontrolled diabetes, hypertension, thyroid disease, congestive heart failure, inflammatory arthritis, multiple sclerosis, sepsis, acute illnesses, and fevers
- Large abdominal or inguinal hernias
- Hemorrhoids
- Unstable or acute injury to joints, ligaments, or tendons
- Severe dementia or balance disturbance
- Acute alcohol or drug intoxication
- Acute retinal bleeding or detachment
- Recent ophthalmologic surgery (laser, cataract extraction, retinal, or glaucoma surgery)

If you cannot safely weight train because of any of these conditions, discuss safe alternative forms of exercise with your physician.

Exercises to Avoid if at Risk for Osteoporosis

If you are at risk for or have osteoporosis, you should not perform certain weight training exercises. Any exercise that involves bending (flexion) or turning of the spine against resistance may increase the risk of compression fractures of vertebrae in the chest region (Singh 2000). Therefore, avoid bending over to lift weights, and do not perform curl-ups with the feet hooked under an exercise bar or the sofa while raising the chest all the way to the knees. Instead of bending over to lift a weight, lower your body by bending at the knees while keeping the back straight. At many gyms the hand weights are located on an upright rack, so use care when lifting them. When doing abdominal crunches, or curl-ups, lie on your back, and bend your knees while keeping your feet flat on the floor. Use your abdominal muscles to do the curl-ups without bending your spine. Other exercises to avoid include leg presses on a machine, toe raises on a machine, and squats with a bar resting on the shoulders (Singh 2000).

Weight Training Safety

Proper breathing is important during resistance training. Working muscles need oxygen to resist fatigue and prevent injury (Hales and Zartman 2001). In strength training, the most common mistake is to hold your breath as you strain to lift a weight. Doing so reduces the blood flow back to your heart, causing you to feel faint or dizzy (Fahey, Insel, and Roth 2003). Be sure to exhale during the contraction and inhale when the muscles are relaxing. When performing a set of repetitions, exhale during the lift and inhale each time the weight is lowered. Rest periods between sets should be two to three minutes for multiple-joint exercises (e.g., bench press, leg press) that involve a heavy load, whereas a one- to two-minute rest period is adequate for single-joint exercises, such as biceps curls (ACSM 2002).

Use available mirrors while performing strength training to help you keep your body in proper alignment during the exercises. Keep your hips, shoulders, and knees in the same vertical plane, and avoid arching your back during any lift. Learning and using correct form are important parts of the early stages of a resistance training program. Sensible guidelines for weight training are provided in the sidebar on this page.

Avoiding overtraining is another important safety guideline. Resist the urge to get in shape and build or rebuild muscle in one week. Muscles need at least 48 hours to recover from progressive resistance training (ACSM 2001). If you find that you really enjoy strength training and want to perform strength training workouts more frequently than twice a week, plan to alternate the muscle groups you would be working. For example, you could exercise your shoulders, chest, arms, and upper back on Mondays and Thursdays, and then work on your abdominals, thighs, hamstrings, and calves on Tuesdays and Fridays. Remember to create a balanced overall fitness program that includes cardiorespiratory and flexibility activities on the days you are not strength training. Additionally, the workout variety during the week will help maintain your enthusiasm for your total fitness program in the long run.

Sensible Guidelines for Resistance Training

The following resistance training guidelines are offered to increase your safety and satisfaction (Graves and Franklin 2001):

▸ No matter what your overall goal may be, your personal strength program should safely develop or maintain your muscular fitness so you can live an active and independent life.

▸ If you have never performed any weightlifting exercises, initially seek the advice and supervision of qualified fitness personnel. For specific information on how to select a health/fitness facility or a personal trainer, see chapter 8. In addition, ACSM has three helpful brochures, "Selecting and Effectively Using a Personal Trainer," "Selecting and Effectively Using a Health/Fitness Facility," and "Selecting and Effectively Using Free Weights." To obtain these brochures, go to www.acsm.org/health+fitness/brochures.htm.

▸ At the beginning of a strength training program, especially if you have been inactive previously, give the muscles, tendons, and ligaments time to adapt to the work. Use minimum levels of resistance (about 50 to 60 percent of the maximum weight you can lift). You should be able to complete 12 reps without straining.

▸ To avoid injury and receive the maximum benefit of the exertion, you should perform each weightlifting exercise correctly and with proper lifting technique. This means that you should lift and lower the weight in a slow, controlled manner whether you are using free weights or machines.

▸ Use a weight or resistance that you can lift for at least 8 repetitions per set.

▸ At first, overload by increasing the number of repetitions (from 8 to 12), then increase the amount of weight, or resistance.

▸ Avoid lifting when you are sick or in pain (from strained or sprained muscles) or have inflamed joints.

▸ Avoid overtraining. Although you will be eager to see quick results, two strength training sessions per week will produce increases in muscular fitness and decreases in body fat.

The major risks of strength training include musculoskeletal injury and cardiovascular events (Singh 2000). Carefully following the previous guidelines will reduce the potential for these two problems.

Anatomy of a Strength Training Session

A well-structured PRT workout includes a warm-up before the resistance training. After the resistance training, you should also include a cool-down. This section explains the elements of a complete strength workout.

Warm-Up

Similar to your preparation for a cardiorespiratory workout, a warm-up is needed before a strength training workout. Walk briskly, jog, cycle, or perform light calisthenics for 10 to 20 minutes to warm up the muscles and elevate the heart rate. Be sure to warm up the same muscles and joints that you will use during the workout.

Lifting Phase

Several considerations need to be made for the actual lifting phase of your program. You need to decide on the duration of your workout, arrange your chosen exercises in the most effective order, ensure proper lifting technique, and include exercises for opposing muscles to avoid imbalances.

Targeting a Reasonable Duration

Performing one or two exercises for each muscle group is sufficient for a workout (Willoughby 2001). It takes about 20 minutes to complete one set of weight training exercises for the six major muscle groups (chest, shoulders, arms, back, abdomen, and legs). As your muscular fitness and weightlifting skill increase, your resistance training program can incorporate up to three sets of exercises in a 45-minute session (Willoughby 2001).

Order of Exercises

Opinions differ as to the correct order of performing strength training exercises, but for optimal safety we recommend exercising the large muscles first, followed by the smaller muscles or muscle groups. This allows for accommodation of the high intensity or greater weight levels needed for bone building in perimenopausal and postmenopausal women.

For older adults, the ACSM (2001) recommends weight training programs emphasizing multiple-joint exercises (using more than one joint such as the bench press or leg press). Specific ACSM advice for novice to advanced strength training includes the following recommendations (ACSM 2002, 368):

- In a workout for all major muscle groups, exercise large muscle groups before small muscle groups, and perform multiple-joint exercises before single-joint exercises.

- For workouts focusing on upper body muscles one day and lower body muscles another day, train large muscle groups before performing small muscle group exercises, and perform multiple-joint exercises before single-joint exercises.

- If training individual muscle groups, do multiple-joint exercises before single-joint exercises and higher-intensity exercises before lower-intensity exercises.

Lifting Technique

When performing a repetition, control the movement and the resistance. Slower speeds of lifting and lowering the weight increase the tension of the muscle and decrease the possibility of injury (Westcott and Baechle 1998). For untrained individuals, a slower lowering phase is recommended to effectively work the muscles. Therefore, complete each repetition in six seconds: two seconds to lift and four seconds to lower (ACSM 2002). With intermediate strength training skills, use a moderate velocity for strength training: one to two seconds to lift and one to two seconds to lower (ACSM 2002).

Training Opposing Muscles

For your strength training routine, remember to stimulate the opposing muscles, those on the opposite side of the joint, to avoid developing a strength imbalance (Westcott and Baechle 1998). For example, you should work the muscles in front of the thighs (quadriceps) and in back of the thighs (hamstrings), the muscles in front and back of the arms (biceps and triceps), and the abdominal muscles and lower back muscles.

During a workout, you might start with leg exercises, then proceed to upper body muscles (chest, back, and shoulders) and the upper arms (biceps and triceps). You should finish with exercises for your midsection because these muscles stabilize the spine and should not be exhausted until the last part of the strength workout (Westcott and Baechle 1998). Other than exercising the large muscles first and the midsection last, the specific order for progressive resistance exercises is your preference.

Cool-Down

After completing your strength training workout, be sure to walk or cycle to help your heart and muscles make the transition from strenuous exercises to normal activity. At least 5 minutes are needed for the cool-down activity. In addition, gently stretching the muscles that were targeted during the workout is helpful.

Assessing Muscular Strength

To assess your general strength, the YMCA leg extension test is a good place to start because it appraises muscular strength for ages 50 to 79 in relation to your body weight (Westcott and Baechle 1998). On the leg extension (leg press) machine, begin with an amount that is 25 percent of your body weight and complete 10 repetitions using the following directions (Westcott and Baechle 1998, 15):

1. Lift the weight by extending your legs (without locking your knees) within two seconds.
2. Hold the position briefly.
3. Lower the weight in four seconds, almost allowing the stack of weights to touch before beginning the next rep.

Rest for two minutes and repeat the procedure using a weight that is 35 percent of your body weight. If you're able, continue alternating two-minute rests with weight loads that increase by 10 percent until you reach the heaviest weight you can lift 10 times with good lifting form. Divide this weight load by your body weight to determine your strength score (see table 4.1 for your leg fitness classification).

Table 4.1   YMCA Leg Extension Test Score Categories for Women

Strength fitness	Age 50-59	Age 60-69	Age 70-79
Low	34 or lower	29 or lower	24 or lower
Below average	35-44	30-39	25-34
Average	45-54	40-49	35-44
Above average	55-64	50-59	45-54
High	65 or higher	60 or higher	55 or higher

Example: 10 reps completed with 60 lb
60 lb divided by 120 lb = .50 = Above average for 70-year-old female

Reprinted, by permission, from W.L. Westcott and T.R. Baechle, 1998, *Strength training past 50* (Champaign, IL: Human Kinetics), 16.

If you do not have access to a leg press machine, the leg squat is a good option for a test of general strength. Leg squats need no equipment or computations. To perform the leg squat test, follow these procedures (Westcott and Baechle 1998, 17):

1. With feet shoulder-width apart, stand 6 to 12 inches in front of a chair.
2. Fold your arms across your chest, and keep your back straight while you slowly squat until your buttocks touch the seat of the chair.
3. Keep your knees directly above your toes during the squat.
4. The entire leg squat should take four seconds to lower to touch the chair seat and two seconds to return to standing. Do not bounce on the chair seat.
5. Perform the leg squats at this pace until you cannot maintain proper form or until you feel muscle pain. In table 4.2, find your fitness category in the row that intersects your age and the number of squats you completed.

These strength evaluations are meant to be used as markers when beginning a resistance training program. Remember that you are working on gaining or maintaining strength, so be positive about your fitness goal. Do not let low assessments prevent you from starting your weight training program.

One-repetition maximum tests (1RM) are often used to assess muscular strength in competitive athletics or during fitness classes. The 1RM tests determine the greatest amount of weight you can lift one time for a given exercise. For the purpose of establishing a general exercise program, it is not vital to determine your 1RM. If you do desire to determine your 1RM for various exercises, see the sidebar on page 70.

Table 4.2 Leg Squat Test Score Categories for Women

Strength fitness	Age 50-59	Age 60-69	Age 70-79
Low	6-8 reps	3-5 reps	0-2 reps
Below average	9-11 reps	6-8 reps	3-5 reps
Average	12-14 reps	9-11 reps	6-8 reps
Above average	15-17 reps	12-14 reps	9-11 reps
High	18-20 reps	15-17 reps	12-14 reps

Reprinted, by permission, from W.L. Westcott and T.R. Baechle, 1998, *Strength training past 50* (Champaign, IL: Human Kinetics), 19.

Directions for 1RM Tests

If you choose to perform the 1RM test, start with a weight level that you can lift easily. Rest two to three minutes after lifting that weight, then increase it by 5 to 10 pounds for the next trial (ACSM 2001). Repeat this process until you reach the last weight level you can successfully lift with proper form. The 1RM test measures dynamic strength and is performed with the same free weights or weight machine used during regular strength training workouts (ACSM 2001). To assess your progress, conduct the 1RM test every three months.

Assessing Muscular Endurance

You can determine dynamic muscular endurance in several ways. One method is to perform the maximum number of repetitions possible with a selected percentage of your 1RM or using a set percentage of your body weight (ACSM 2001). Most often, the maximum number of curl-ups, push-ups, pull-ups, or chin-ups you can perform is used to calculate your level of muscular endurance. If your muscular fitness is below average or your weight is above average, these calisthenics can be more a test of muscular strength than of endurance (ACSM 2001). Don't discount calisthenic-type exercises just because they have been around for a while. They still can improve your initial muscular endurance.

To check the number of push-ups or curl-ups you can do, use the following information (Canadian Society for Exercise Physiology [CSEP] 2003, 7-40):

• Push-ups: The starting position for a modified (knee) push-up is lying on your stomach with your legs together. Your hands should be under your shoulders and pointing forward. Using your knees as the pivot point, push up until your arms are straight. Proper technique includes keeping the upper body straight and keeping the knees, lower legs, and feet on the mat. (Your toes are pointed so that your ankles and the tops of your feet are touching the mat.) Return to the beginning position. During the "down" phase, your abdomen and thighs should not touch the mat. This counts as one push-up. Exhale during the pushing up phase. Using good form, perform as many push-ups as you can without straining or stopping. Compare your number with rankings in table 4.3.

Table 4.3   Fitness Norms for Push-Ups for Women

Performance ranking	Age 30-39	Age 40-49	Age 50-59	Age 60-69
Excellent	27 or higher	24 or higher	21 or higher	17 or higher
Very good	20-26	15-23	11-20	12-16
Good	13-19	11-14	7-10	5-11
Fair	8-12	5-10	2-6	2-4
Needs improvement	7 or lower	4 or lower	1 or lower	1 or lower

Source: The Canadian Physical Activity, Fitness & Lifestyle Approach: CSEP-Health & Fitness Program's Health-Related Appraisal and Counselling Strategy (3rd edition), © 2003. Reprinted with permission from the Canadian Society for Exercise Physiology.

• Curl-ups: To perform a partial curl-up, lie on your back on a mat with knees bent to 90 degrees and feet flat on the mat. Your arms should be extended along the sides of your body. Have a helper place a strip of masking tape at the point where your fingertips touch the mat. Place another piece of tape 3.9 inches (10 cm) beyond the first strip of tape. One complete curl-up involves lifting your shoulders off the mat to touch the second piece of tape with your fingers and returning your back to the mat. Exhale during the curl-up phase. Your palms and heels must maintain contact with the mat during the curl-up. Each curl-up should take approximately two seconds. To assist with maintaining the correct cadence, you can set a metronome to 50 beats per minute (so you would curl up on one click and then return your shoulders to the mat on the next click to complete one curl-up). Perform as many as possible at this rate without stopping, to a maximum of 25 in one minute. Use table 4.4 to determine your abdominal fitness level.

Table 4.4   *Fitness Norms for Partial Curl-Ups for Women*

Performance ranking	Age 30-39	Age 40-49	Age 50-59	Age 60-69
Excellent	25	25	25	25
Very good	19-24	19-24	19-24	17-24
Good	10-18	11-18	10-18	8-16
Fair	6-9	4-10	6-9	3-7
Needs improvement	5 or lower	3 or lower	5 or lower	2 or lower

Source: The Canadian Physical Activity, Fitness & Lifestyle Approach: CSEP-Health & Fitness Program's Health-Related Appraisal and Counselling Strategy (3rd edition), © 2003. Reprinted with permission from the Canadian Society for Exercise Physiology.

Exercise Progression

When you begin a strength training program, learn the proper lifting techniques for each exercise and muscle group. Those who are at a lower fitness level should first master any new resistance exercise using only gravity or body weight, then progress to exercise bands, dumbbells, or weight machines (Hyatt 1996). If possible, practice in front of a mirror, and use the lightest weight possible while concentrating on correct breathing (exhaling during the lift) and keeping the body properly aligned (head, shoulders, hips, and ankles in line). Use a small notebook or strength training chart to monitor the resistance used for each exercise. (See table 4.8 at the end of this chapter.)

As your muscular strength increases, so will the number of repetitions you can perform at an initial level of resistance. We recommend starting with a low weight you can easily lift for 10 to 12 repetitions. If you are beginning a resistance training program, there is no such thing as too light a weight. The communication between the brain and the muscle is the first step in gaining strength. Once you learn the proper way to perform the exercise, you can begin to increase the resistance.

When you can correctly lift 12 reps at a given resistance during two consecutive workouts, you should add two to five pounds to this exercise. This method, known as a double progressive program of increasing the repetitions and then the resistance, helps prevent unnecessary soreness and overtraining injuries (Westcott and Baechle 1998). With the new weight, start building the number of repetitions back up to 12, using a slow to moderate lifting velocity. You can progress from one to three sets for each exercise, lifting 8 to 12 repetitions of each (ACSM 2002). To help you get started, five easy steps to beginning strength exercises are provided in the sidebar on page 73.

Five Easy Steps to Beginning Strength Exercises

1. Make a commitment.
   - Exercise will take some time and effort.
   - Expect to strength train 20 to 45 minutes two or three times each week.
   - You may be a little sore the first week, but it will pass.

2. Find a good resource.
   - It could be a personal trainer or a good book (including examples given in this chapter).
   - Try the National Institute on Aging's guide to exercise (1-800-222-2225).
   - Learn 8 to 10 exercises to strengthen all the major muscle groups.

3. Develop a routine.
   - Perform 8 to 15 repetitions (one complete "lift and relax" cycle) for each set and two to three sets of each exercise.
   - If you cannot do at least 8 repetitions, the weight is too heavy.
   - Breathe once for each repetition; always move the weight slowly.
   - Rest two minutes between sets, or do an exercise with a different muscle group.
   - Your whole workout should take less than 45 minutes.

4. Progress as you improve.
   - If you exceed 15 repetitions, the weight is too light; gradually increase the resistance.
   - At first you will be increasing the weight every week or so.

5. Rest and grow.
   - Do not do strengthening exercise routines on two consecutive days.
   - Rest to give your muscles a chance to recuperate.
   - You will become much stronger—probably 25 to 100 percent stronger in each muscle.
   - Research shows the biggest improvements are in the first few months.

Reprinted with permission of the American College of Sports Medicine. ©American College of Sports Medicine. www.acsm.org

Using Machines and Free Weights

It is your choice whether to use machines or free weights or a combination of the two. There are advantages and disadvantages to both. As you read this section, think about your strength needs, your personal preferences, and whether you prefer to conduct your weight training sessions at home or in a fitness center.

Weight Machines

If you are a beginner, there are several advantages to using weightlifting machines. A major advantage is that they don't require a great deal of skill or strength to use. You select the resistance or weight you can comfortably lift. Another convenience is that the increments of weight increases can be fairly small, helping you match the resistance to the amount you can lift. If your strength in a group of muscles is not particularly high, machines allow greater control in the direction of movement, thereby increasing the safety of the exercise (Graves and Franklin 2001). Machines are usually designed to provide more support for the lower back than occurs with the use of free weights (Graves and Franklin 2001), but it is important to adjust the machine to fit your body height and the length of your arms, legs, and torso.

No matter what your experience level, some weight training exercises are more easily performed on a machine (e.g., hip adduction) (Hoeger and Hoeger 2002). Weight machines are also extremely useful for rehabilitating joints after an injury or surgery. Safety considerations for using weight machines include the following recommendations:

- Read the directions and study any pictures on the machines so you can perform the exercise correctly. Adjust the machine to fit your height and arm or leg length as appropriate. Secure all supports or adjustable items before you start to lift. If it is your first time using weight machines, request in advance that a staff person demonstrate the proper use of each machine.

- Many people use the machines in succession. To avoid bare skin contact with dirty or wet vinyl surfaces, use a towel on the machine where you will sit or lie. After using a machine, wipe your sweat from the seat and handles.

- Pay attention to safety when using the machines. Stay away from moving parts of other machines, and always fully insert the pin in the weight stack.

The ACSM recommends that older adults may initially begin with weight machines and then progress to free weights as they gain strength training experience (ACSM 2002).

Free Weights

Free weights are not connected to a weight machine. They include the weight plates that slide onto each end of a bar (to create a barbell), hand weights (dumbbells), and ankle weights.

The use of free weights also has advantages and disadvantages. On the positive side, they are relatively inexpensive, can be used at home, and come in varying weight increments. Additionally, there is an almost infinite amount of resistance exercises possible to work specific muscle groups when using free weights. The disadvantages of free weights include that they require more balance, coordination, and skill. The risk of injury from a falling weight is greater when using free weights. For safety, a spotter is needed when using barbells. Calluses and blisters are more common with free weight use, so wearing weightlifting gloves with padded palms is recommended.

The most important thing is to incorporate progressive resistance training into your overall fitness program. Whether you opt to use free weights at home or weight machines at a fitness center (perhaps including a combination of both), a well-planned strength program will make your transition into or through menopause easier and healthier.

Strength Training Exercises

This section includes basic strength training exercises used when exercising with weight machines and free weights. As you read through these exercises, use the chart at the end of the chapter to note the exercises you want to include in your PRT program.

Machine Training Exercises

What areas of your body need strengthening? Where would you like to see better muscle definition or tone? The following exercise descriptions identify which muscles will be worked and explain how to perform each exercise on weight machines commonly found at fitness centers. Strength machines will vary, so follow the directions on each one to perform the exercise correctly. Adjust the seat to fit your height, and change machine arms to fit your range of motion. Use lap belts if the machines have them.

LEG PRESS

Works the muscles on the front and back of the thigh and the buttocks: quadriceps, hamstrings, and gluteals

Start with the knees flexed at 90 degrees or less, with feet flat on the foot pads. Knees and feet should be in line with the hips. Exhale during the press. Push your feet and legs forward until they are nearly extended. Do not lock your knees. Slowly return to the starting position without banging the weights.

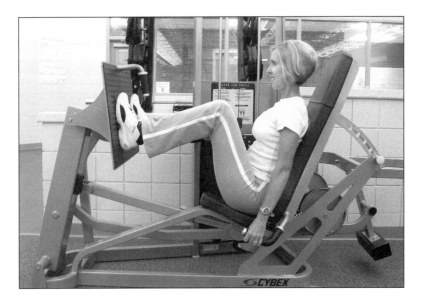

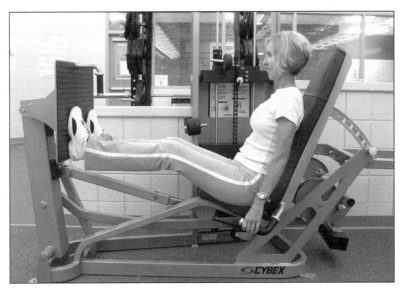

CHEST PRESS

Works the upper body muscles that push: pectoralis major

Sit with your back against the seat pads. Grip the bar handles with your palms facing away from the body. Exhale and push the handles forward until the arms are extended. Inhale while returning the handles to the starting position.

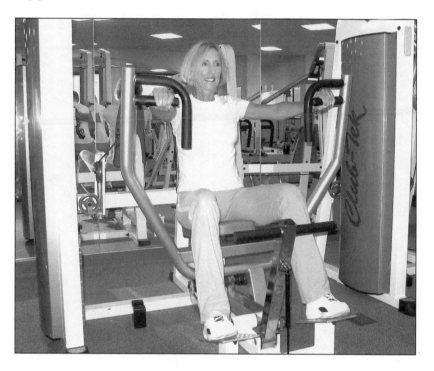

COMPOUND ROW

Works the upper body muscles that pull: latissimus dorsi and back

This exercise is also called the seated row. Move the seat so your shoulders are level with the machine handles. Press your chest against the chest pad and grasp the handles. Exhale while slowly pulling the handles back toward your chest. Inhale while returning to the starting position.

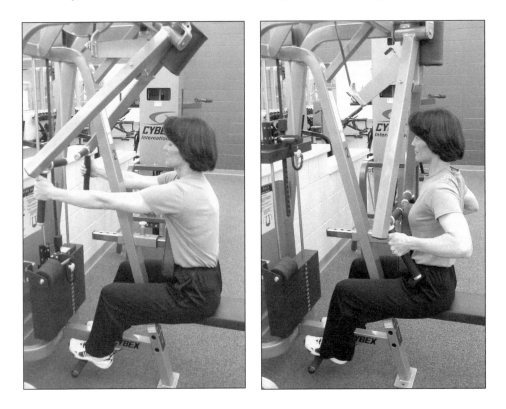

PULL-UP AND CHIN-UP

Work the biceps and latissimus dorsi muscles

On this machine, the more weight on the weight stack, the less weight you will lift as you complete the exercise. For pull-ups, grasp the bar with palms facing away from the body (figure *a*). Palms should face your body when performing chin-ups (figure *b*). Lower your body until your arms are extended. Begin the exercise from this position, exhaling as you pull your chin above the bar and inhaling as you lower your body.

Some machines require you to stand during the exercise, while others use a kneeling position. Compare the pull-up using an overhead grip (figure *a*) with the chin-up using an underhand grip on a kneeling machine (figure *b*).

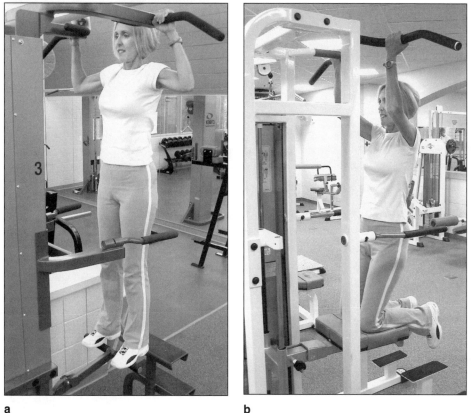

a   b

ABDOMINAL CURL

Works the abdominal muscles: rectus abdominis

Position the chest pad above the breasts, and rest your hands on your thighs. Exhale and slowly bend forward until your back is flexed and your abdominal muscles are tight. Inhale while gradually returning to the starting position.

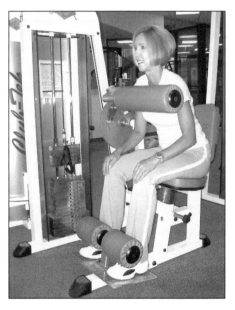

BACK EXTENSION

Works the lower back muscles: erector spinae

Sit against the back of the seat and rest your hands lightly on your legs or cross your arms on your chest. Exhale and press your back and shoulders backward against the pad until your back is nearly straight. Inhale while returning to the beginning position.

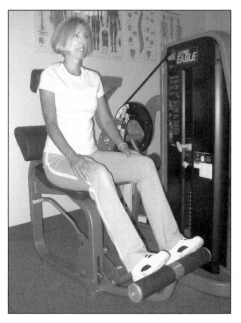

LAT PULL-DOWN

Works the latissimus dorsi, biceps, and back muscles

Adjust the seat height and extend your arms overhead to grasp the bar.
Your palms are facing forward, with hands at least shoulder-width apart.
Exhale and pull the bar down to your collarbone (by tucking your chin
to allow the bar to freely pass in front of your face). Inhale and return to
the beginning position.

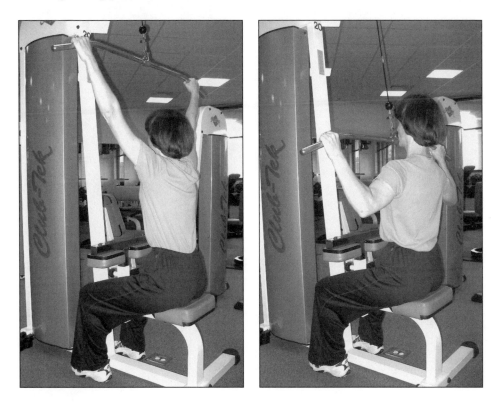

BICEPS CURL

Works the muscles on the front of the upper arm: biceps

Position the seat height so the fully outstretched arms are supported by the pad. Keep the back straight and grasp the handles palm up. Exhale as you pull the bar to a vertical position.

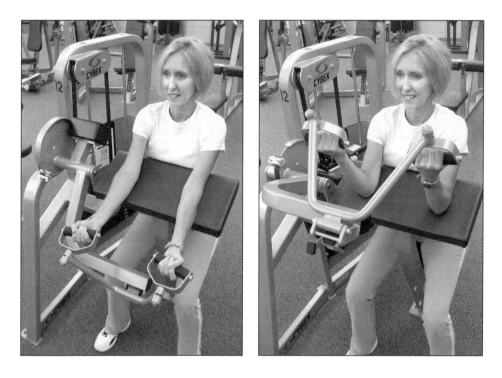

TRICEPS PRESS

Works the muscles on the back of the upper arm: triceps

Move the seat height so your upper arms are resting flat against the arm pad. Grasp the handles and push forward until the arms are straight, exhaling while you push. Keep your back straight during this exercise.

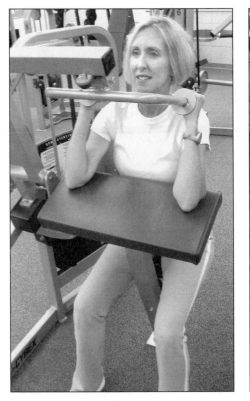 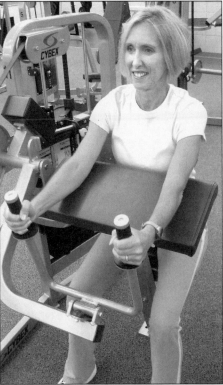

HIP ADDUCTION

Works the inner thigh muscles: hip adductors

Sit with your back pressed against the seat pad. Your knees should be on the outside of the knee pads and your feet and ankles in the machine's supports. Adjust the lever so your legs are spread comfortably apart. Exhale as you press your knees together during the exercise, and inhale during the return.

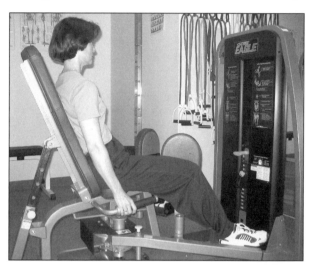

HIP ABDUCTION

Works the outer thigh muscles: hip abductors

Sit squarely in the seat with your back and shoulders against the seat back. Your knees will be on the inside knee pads, with your ankles and feet resting in the machine supports. Exhale as you push your knees apart during the exercise, and inhale during the return.

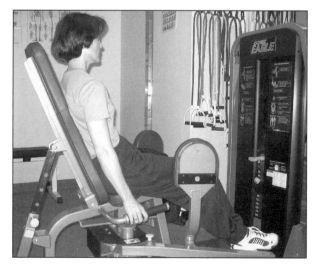

Free Weight Training Exercises

Free weights put you in charge during the exercise, so using a mirror will help you perform the movement correctly. It is uncommon for women to select free weights that are too heavy; it is more likely that your choice will be too light to be therapeutically useful (Singh 2000). Add the free weight exercises you will perform on the strength training chart at the end of the chapter.

If you are strength training at home, you can use a variety of items for weights, depending on your level of muscular fitness. Full cans of soup are a cheap and readily available form of resistance, weighing between 10 and 16 ounces. Small hand dumbbells range in weight from 1 to 10 pounds. A plastic gallon jug, filled with water, weighs about 8 pounds. You can use any of these homemade weights during upper body exercises in one to three sets of 8 to 12 repetitions, resting one to two minutes between sets (Fleck and Kraemer 1998).

Concentrate on breathing correctly and on properly performing the lift through the full range of motion. When lifting during some exercises, you can stand or sit. Realize that a few more calories are burned while performing upper body exercises when standing. Keep your torso stationary when performing the strength exercises.

DUMBBELL BENCH PRESS

Works the upper body muscles that push: pectoralis major

Lie on a sturdy bench with knees bent and feet flat on the bench. Head, shoulders, back, and buttocks must maintain contact with the bench during the bench press. Hold the dumbbells with palms facing up. Exhale and push the dumbbells up until arms are straight.

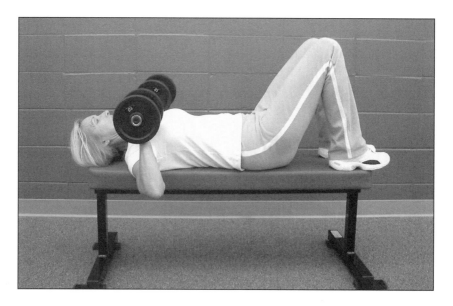

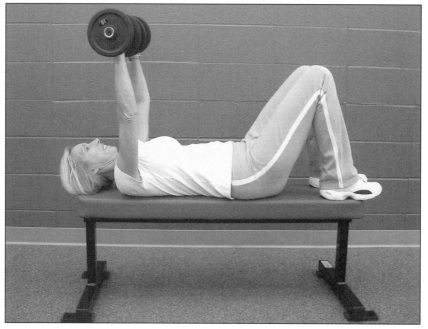

DUMBBELL ONE-ARM ROW

Works the upper body muscles that pull: latissimus dorsi and back

One dumbbell and a bench are needed for this exercise. Stand on the right side of the bench; place your left knee and the palm of your left hand on the bench, keeping the left arm straight. Hold the dumbbell in your right hand, with the palm toward the bench. Stand on your right leg and keep your back straight. Exhale and pull the dumbbell toward the side of your chest. Inhale as you return to the starting position. Continue with the other arm, changing leg positions on the bench.

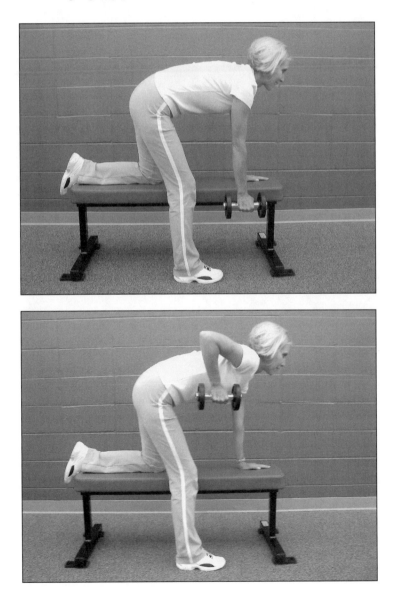

SEATED ARM RAISE

Works the shoulder muscles: deltoids

Sit in a sturdy chair with a back. Your feet should be flat on the floor. With your arms hanging at your sides, hold the dumbbells with palms facing backward. Exhale and raise the dumbbells to shoulder height, keeping elbows straight. Inhale and lower the dumbbells to the starting position.

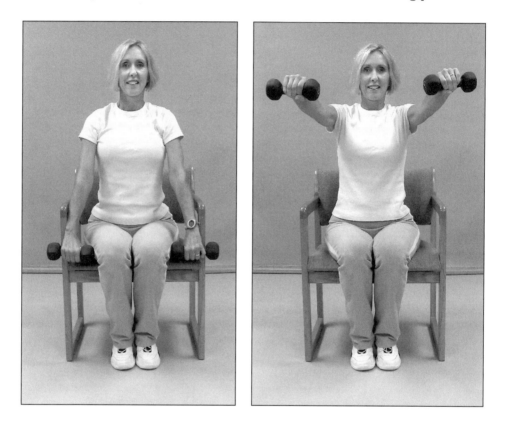

SEATED ARM ABDUCTION

Works the shoulder and upper back muscles

Sit in a chair with feet flat on the floor. Grasp dumbbells with palms turned forward. Keep elbows straight and raise the dumbbells out and away from your sides, touching them as high overhead as possible.

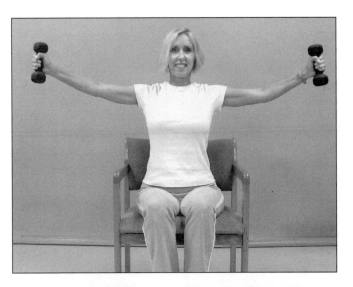

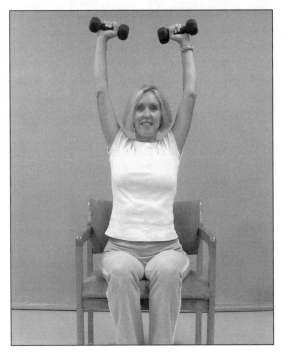

OVERHEAD PRESS

Works the shoulder muscles: deltoids

Sit straight in a chair with your feet flat on the floor. Hold the dumbbells at shoulder height with your palms forward. Bend arms to a 90 degree angle. Exhale and raise both arms overhead until arms are straight and the weights touch. Inhale and return to the starting position.

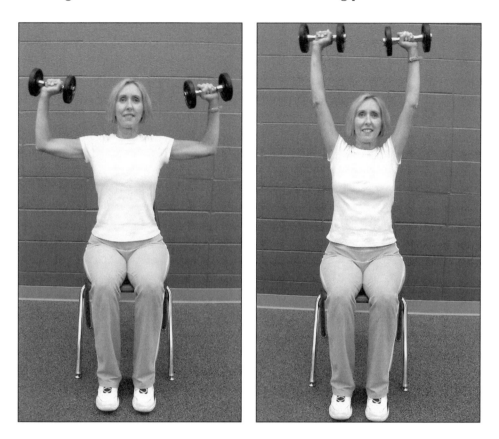

UPRIGHT ROW

Works the shoulder and upper back muscles

Stand tall with feet about 12 inches apart. With palms facing the body, hold the dumbbells at the front of your thighs. Exhale and lift both dumbbells straight up the midline of your body to the height of your collarbone. Your elbows should be sticking out to each side. Inhale and lower the weights to the starting position.

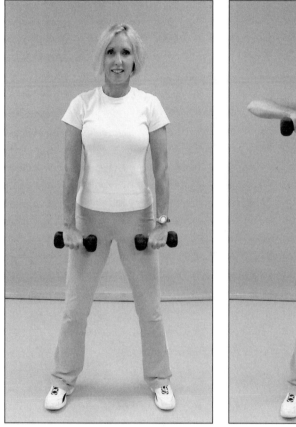 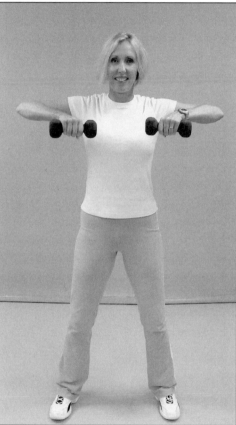

CHEST FLY

Works the chest and pectoral muscles

Lie on your back on the floor, with your knees bent and feet on the floor. With a dumbbell in each hand, extend your arms out to shoulder level. Exhale and lift the weights, using a slight elbow bend to touch the dumbbells in the air directly above your chest. Inhale as you return the dumbbells to the starting position.

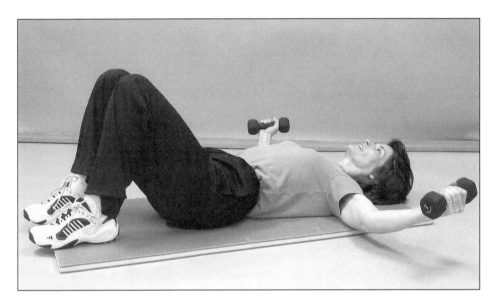

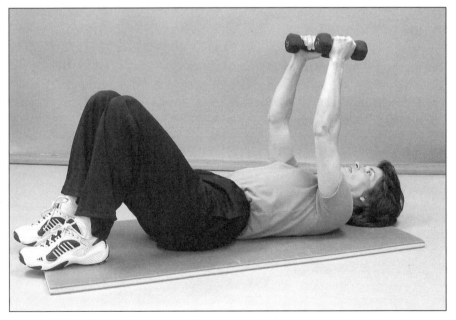

BICEPS CURL

Works the muscles on the front of the upper arm: biceps

Stand tall with feet shoulder-width apart. Hold the dumbbells with the palms facing forward. Bend the elbows and raise both dumbbells toward your shoulders. Exhale during the lift. Inhale and lower both dumbbells to the starting position. This exercise can also be performed in a seated position, as well as by alternating arms. Keep the torso still if alternating arms.

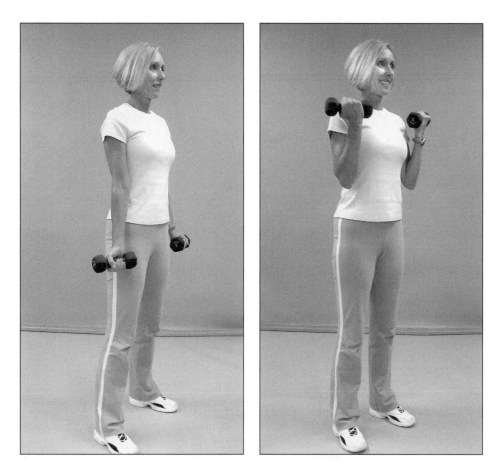

OVERHEAD TRICEPS EXTENSION

Works the muscles on the back of the upper arm: triceps

Stand tall with feet shoulder-width apart. Hold the dumbbell with both hands, and raise both arms over your head. Exhale and lower the dumbbell toward your spine. Inhale and lift the dumbbell to the original position above your head.

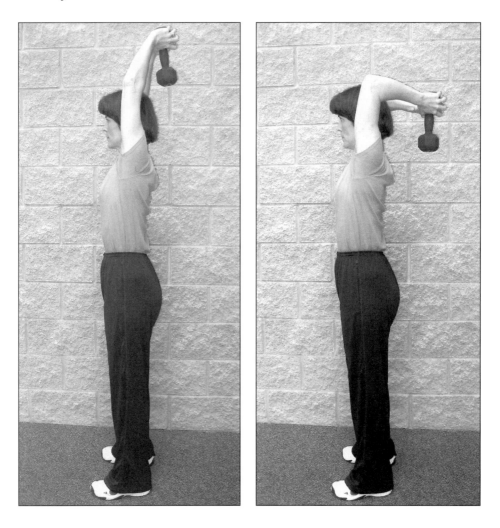

LEG EXTENSION

Works the muscles on the front of the thigh: quadriceps

Ankle weights are needed for this exercise. Sit tall in a chair with feet flat on the floor. Grasp the sides or arms of the chair with your hands. Exhale and raise one lower leg until it is parallel to the floor, with toes pulled back toward the knee. Inhale and lower the leg to the floor. Alternate legs.

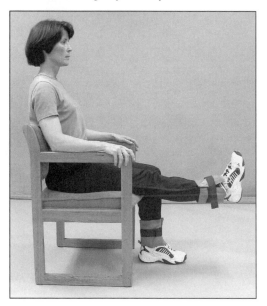

KNEE FLEXION

Works the muscles on the back of the thigh: hamstrings

Wearing ankle weights, stand tall behind a chair. As needed for balance, touch or grasp the chair back. Exhale and bend one knee to raise your foot toward your buttock without moving the thigh. Inhale and lower the leg. Alternate legs.

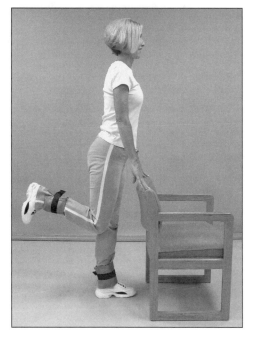

HIP ABDUCTION

Works the muscles on the outside of the thigh

Wearing ankle weights, stand tall with your side to the back of a chair. For balance, touch or grasp the chair back. Exhale and move the outer leg about 8 to 12 inches to the side. Keep the spine in proper alignment, and point the toes forward. Inhale and return the foot to the floor. Alternate legs.

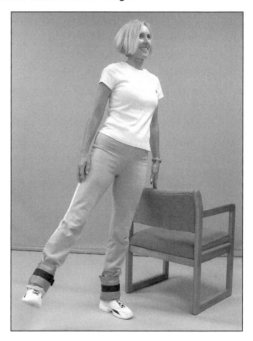

HIP EXTENSION

Works the hamstrings, back of the thighs, and the muscles in the buttocks

Wearing ankle weights, stand tall behind a chair. For balance, touch or grasp the chair back. Bend forward, exhale, and extend one leg straight out behind you. Raise the leg and foot as high as you can. Inhale and return the foot to the floor. Alternate legs. (To decrease the difficulty, you may perform this exercise without ankle weights.)

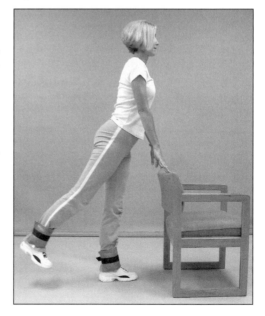

DUMBBELL HEEL RAISE

Works the muscles of the calf: gastrocnemius and soleus

A stable surface two to four inches high is needed for this exercise. Grasp the dumbbells with your palms toward your thighs. Stand with your back straight and head up. The balls of the feet are on the elevated or inclined surface. Keep the weight on the balls of your feet as you lift and lower your heels. Exhale as you raise your heels.

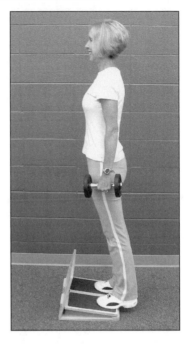

A summary of resistance training exercises that target specific muscle groups of the body is listed in table 4.5 (for anterior muscle groups) and table 4.6 (for posterior muscle groups). Selecting activities from the areas listed will help you design a complete and balanced strength program. For

Table 4.5 Resistance Training Exercises for Anterior (Front Side) Muscle Groups

Muscles	Body area	Exercises
Pectorals	Chest	Chest press, dumbbell bench press, dumbbell chest fly
Deltoids	Shoulders	Overhead press, seated arm raise, seated arm abduction, upright row
Biceps	Front of upper arms	Biceps curl, dumbbell curl
Abdominals	Abdomen	Machine abdominal curl
Quadriceps	Front of thighs	Ankle weight leg extension, leg press

Table 4.6 Resistance Training Exercises for Posterior (Back Side) Muscle Groups

Muscles	Body area	Exercises
Trapezius	Upper back	Compound row, upright row
Triceps	Back of upper arms	Dumbbell overhead triceps extension, machine triceps press
Latissimus dorsi	Underneath armpits to back sides of chest	Lat pull-down, compound row, one-arm row
Erector spinae	Back	Machine back extension
Gluteus maximus	Buttocks	Leg press, hip extension
Hamstrings	Back of thighs	Leg press, ankle weight knee flexion
Gastrocnemius and soleus	Calves	Dumbbell heel raise

more in-depth information on a variety of resistance training procedures, we recommend *Strength Training Past 50* by Wayne L. Westcott and Thomas R. Baechle (1998, Human Kinetics).

Body Weight and Resistance Band Exercises

At times you will not have access to weight machines or free weights, or perhaps you simply desire an alternative strength workout. For these situations, you can use your own body weight as the resistance or use resistance bands. The disadvantage of using your body weight is the amount of resistance cannot be easily adjusted, and strength gains do not occur without adding additional resistance (Corbin et al. 2002).

Calisthenics

You may remember calisthenics as the dreaded exercises of gym class. If so, it's time for an attitude adjustment. These body weight exercises are good for you. Examples of body weight exercises are push-ups, chin-ups, pull-ups, and curl-ups. The following are descriptions of how to properly perform these selected calisthenics.

PULL-UP AND CHIN-UP

Work the biceps and latissimus dorsi muscles

Standing on a step box or bench can help you perform leg-assisted pull-ups and chin-ups until your arms are strong enough to do full pull-ups or chin-ups (see table 4.7, Progression of Body Weight Exercises). When using a step box or bench, grasp the bar with your hands placed slightly wider than your shoulders, and bend your knees until your arms are almost extended. Exhale and use your legs to assist you in the upward movement. Complete the lowering phase with minimal help from your legs.

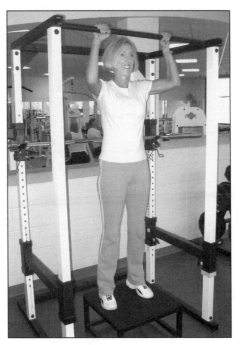

CURL-UP

Works the abdominal muscles: rectus abdominis

These are also called trunk curls, abdominal curls, or crunches. Lie on your back on a towel, mat, or carpet. Bend the knees and keep your feet flat on the floor. Your arms can be extended toward your thighs (for less resistance), or your hands can lightly touch your ears (for greater difficulty). Curl up (raise your head and shoulders) until your shoulder blades leave the floor. Exhale during the curl-up, and roll back to the starting position. For increased difficulty, place your legs on a chair seat or low bench.

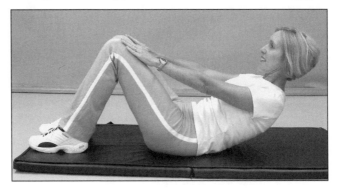

WALL PUSH-UP

Works your chest, pectoral, and triceps muscles

Stand facing a wall and place your palms on the wall at shoulder height. Your palms should be set wider than your shoulders. Keeping your back straight, bend your elbows until your nose almost touches the wall. Exhale as you press away from the wall, and return to the starting position. Moving your feet farther away from the wall will increase the difficulty of this exercise. As you gain more strength in your upper body, progress to bent-knee push-ups on the floor and finally to full push-ups.

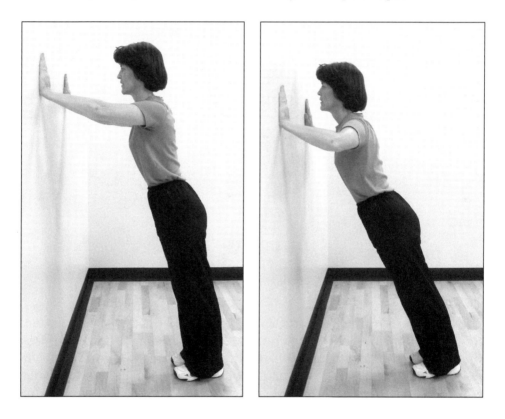

WALL SQUAT

Works the muscles on the front of the thigh: quadriceps

Stand with your back against a wall and your heels about 12 to 18 inches away from the wall (this distance will vary based on your height). Your palms should lightly touch the wall. Exhale and bend at the knees to gently slide down the wall until the knees are over the ankles. Hold this position for several seconds. Inhale and return to a standing position.

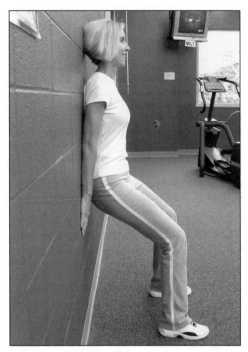

For low levels of initial strength, start with less demanding body weight exercises and progress to greater levels of difficulty (Westcott and Baechle 1998). A progression of body weight exercises is provided in table 4.7.

Table 4.7 *Progression of Body Weight Exercises*

Exercise	Level			
	Easiest	**Medium difficulty**	**Semi-difficult**	**Most difficult**
Push-up	Wall push-up (close to wall)	Wall push-up (farther from wall)	Floor bent-knee push-up	Floor push-up (full extension)
Pull-up	Step box pull-up: lowering only	Step box pull-up: leg assist	Partial pull-up	Full pull-up
Curl-up	Curl-up with bent knees, hands on thighs	Curl-up with bent knees, hands touching ears	Curl-up with lower legs on bench	
Wall squat	Partial wall squat (quarter knee-bends)	Wall squat		

Data from W.L. Westcott and T.R. Baechle, 1998.

Resistance Band Exercises

Resistance bands are made from elastic or rubber and come in assorted lengths and thicknesses to provide varying resistance. Some resistance bands resemble giant rubber bands, and some look like a jump rope made from bungee cord. You will need several resistance bands to exercise your different muscle groups. When traveling, they are light, handy, and versatile.

Almost any free weight movement can be duplicated with resistance bands (Westcott and Baechle 1998). For example, you can perform leg lunges, biceps curls, upright rows, seated chest presses, seated rows, hip abductions, and triceps extensions using resistance bands.

BAND LEG LUNGE

Start in a stride position with one foot in the middle of the band. With arms bent, pull the bands tight. Exhale and perform a lunge, keeping the knee above the ankle on the front leg. Return to the starting position.

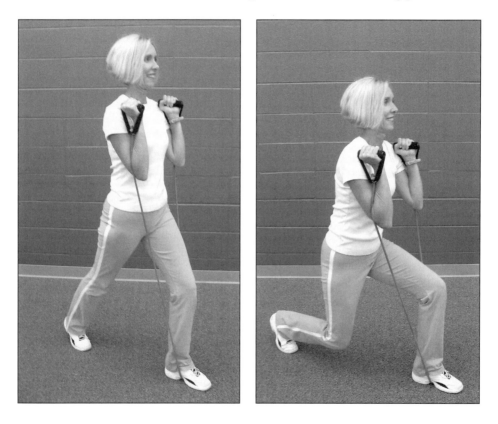

BAND BICEPS CURL AND UPRIGHT ROW

Stand on the resistance band with feet shoulder-width apart. (Refer to the earlier descriptions of these exercises using free weights.) Perform the exercises, exhaling as your muscles contract.

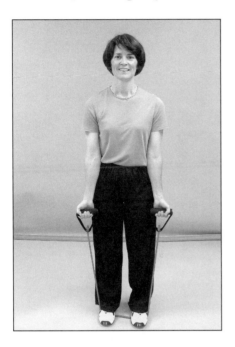

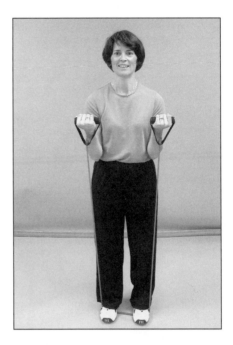

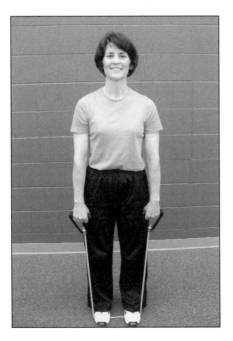

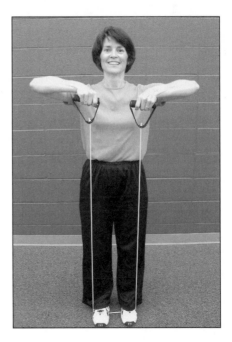

BAND SEATED PRESS

A sturdy chair is needed. The middle of the band is placed at the center of the chair back. Bend your elbows, with hands near your chest. The band should be taut in both your hands. Exhale and push your arms straight out at shoulder height, slowly returning your arms to the starting point.

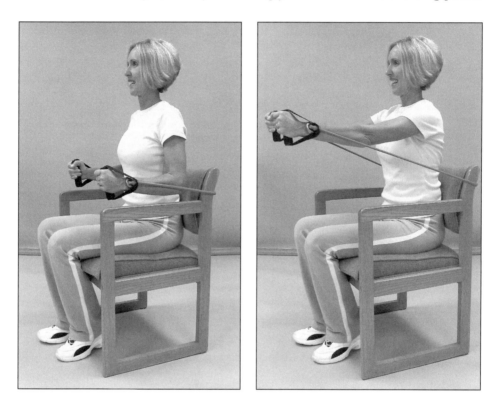

BAND SEATED ROW

Sit on the floor with your back straight and your legs extended in front of you. Make a loose loop with the resistance band and wrap it around the soles of your shoes. Extend your arms in front of you with the ends of the band tight. Exhale and pull your hands toward your chest.

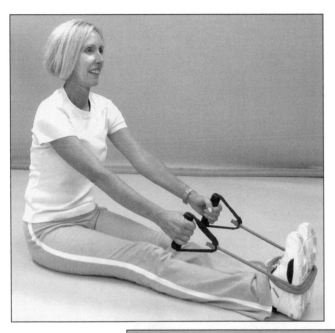

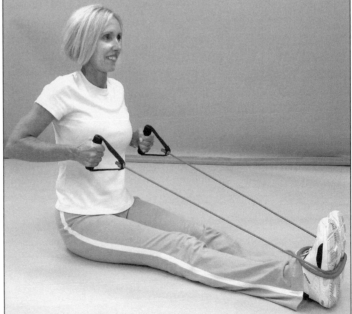

BAND HIP ABDUCTION

Sit on the floor with your back straight and your legs extended in front of you. Make a loose loop with the resistance band and wrap it around the soles of your shoes. Pull the band taut, exhale, and move both your feet away from each other; hold for 4 to 12 seconds.

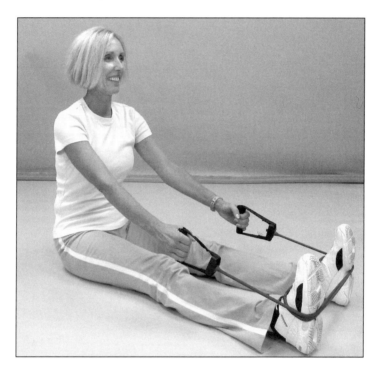

BAND TRICEPS EXTENSION

Hold the band taut in a "zipper stretch position." (See explanation of zipper stretch in chapter 5.) The working arm is the top arm; do not move the lower hand from its position on the lower part of the back. Exhale and extend the working arm straight overhead, then slowly return hand to starting position.

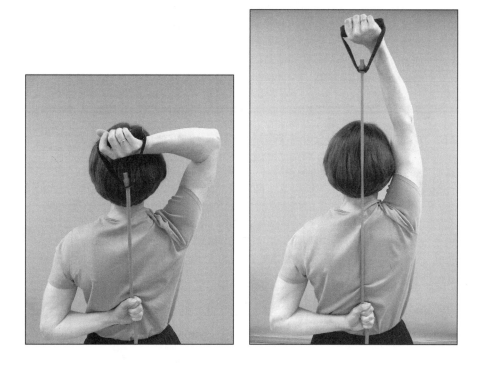

When using the exercise bands, move through the full range of motion in slow, deliberate movements. As with other strength exercises, when you can complete 12 repetitions, move to a stronger band (Westcott and Baechle 1998). Over time, these bands lose their elasticity, so you will need new ones. You can purchase resistance bands at any sporting goods store.

Resuming Resistance Training After a Layoff

Even though you have the best intentions to maintain your resistance training at least two times a week from now on, roadblocks can occur: illness, surgery, or too many demands on your time. Remember that unused muscles may initially experience some soreness if you try to lift at your previous training levels. Expect decreased strength when you start your strength training program again. After a layoff, the ACSM recommends to begin your resistance training program at 50 percent of the intensity (or weight) you were using for each exercise before the cessation of your program (ACSM 2001). Then, progressively rebuild your strength and work to maintain your program, knowing that you do not have to become weaker as you age.

As with any other behavior, when a relapse occurs you should avoid being negative about the situation. Setbacks do happen in life. Use what you learned from this experience to help you avoid similar layoffs in the future (e.g., how can I prevent this from happening again in the future?). Be encouraged that you are resuming your resistance training in order to maintain strong bones and muscles and to prevent unwanted weight gain.

Example of Sally's Resistance Training Program

Sally likes the idea that a weight training program will help her maneuver through the many demands of her elementary teaching position. Like many women, she knows her upper body strength is not as good as it could be. Sally spends much of her day bending over student desks, crouching or squatting to be at eye level with young pupils, and sitting while grading papers. Her specific strength training goals are to accomplish the following:

▸ Increase her arm and shoulder strength

▸ Strengthen the opposing muscles in her abdominal area and lower back

▸ Maintain her leg strength

Sally's schedule and budget don't allow a membership to a gym or fitness center, but she is willing to invest in some free weights (dumbbells, ankle weights), resistance bands, and an exercise mat so she can exercise at home. She knows good deals on these items can be found at garage sales, in the want ads, and at preowned sporting goods stores. Initially, Sally plans to do weight training on the days she is not doing her cardiorespiratory workout. After her warm-up, Sally performs the following exercises: wall squats, hip extensions, hip abductions, knee extensions, heel raises, push-ups, dumbbell bench presses, dumbbell one-arm rows, upright rows, biceps curls, triceps extensions, and abdominal crunches on her mat. She records the weights, number of reps, and number of sets for each exercise during her strength workouts on table 4.8.

Table 4.8   Progressive Resistance Exercise Chart

Use the chart below to plan and monitor your strength conditioning program. First, consider your muscular fitness goal. Is it to increase strength, endurance, or overall fitness? Select the areas of the body to be exercised, using 8 to 10 exercises. Use this chart as you complete your strength workout.

Body area to exercise	Specific exercise (select one per body area)	Number of reps	Number of sets	Amount of weight or band color	Date
Chest	Machine chest press				
	Dumbbell bench press				
	Dumbbell chest fly				
	Band seated chest press				
	Push-up (wall or floor)				
Shoulders	Dumbbell seated arm raise				
	Dumbbell seated arm abduction				
	Dumbbell overhead press				
	Dumbbell or band upright row				
Arms (biceps)	Machine biceps curl				
	Dumbbell or band biceps curl				
	Chin-up				
Arms (triceps)	Machine triceps press				
	Dumbbell overhead triceps extension				
	Band triceps extension				

From *Action Plan for Menopause* by Barbara Bushman and Janice Clark Young, 2005, Champaign, IL: Human Kinetics.

(continued)

Table 4.8 *(continued)*

Back	Machine lat pull-down				
	Machine compound row				
	Dumbbell one-arm row				
	Band seated row				
	Pull-up				
Back (lower)	Machine back extension				
Hip (thigh)	Machine leg press				
	Ankle weight hip extension				
	Band leg lunge				
Leg (quadriceps)	Ankle weight leg extension				
	Wall squat				
Leg (hamstrings)	Ankle weight knee flexion				
Inner thigh	Machine hip adduction				
Outer thigh	Machine hip abduction				
	Band hip abduction				
Calf	Dumbbell heel raise				
Abdomen	Machine abdominal curl				
	Curl-up				

From *Action Plan for Menopause* by Barbara Bushman and Janice Clark Young, 2005, Champaign, IL: Human Kinetics.

Summary

After reading this chapter, take some time to consider how a progressive resistance training program can help you, from perimenopause into menopause. Do you want to maintain your bone density and avoid future osteoporosis and fractures? Wouldn't you love to look great while possessing more toned muscles and less body fat? If you can answer yes to any of these questions, then it is time to begin planning how to use the information in this chapter to regain, maintain, or increase your muscular strength. Your progressive resistance program should be specific to your physical needs, personal lifestyle, and present fitness goals. The individual strength programs we (the authors) use are not identical. One runs while the other swims for cardiorespiratory workouts; therefore, our focus in strength training is somewhat different. Find a time in your schedule when you can perform strength training exercises for 20 to 45 minutes at least two times a week. Select the exercises that fit your needs, and then begin the transformation into the strength goddess you always wanted to become.

ACTION PLAN:
STRENGTHENING POWERFUL WOMEN

☐ Follow safety guidelines for resistance training:
- Warm up before lifting.
- Perform each exercise properly.

☐ Evaluate your present strength:
- Select exercises to target areas needing improved strength.
- Select exercises to maintain areas with good strength.

☐ Determine training frequency and location (home or fitness center).

☐ Select specific resistance exercises to progress toward your strength goals.

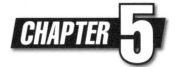

CHAPTER 5

STRETCHING AND LENGTHENING MUSCLES

Although flexibility is not critical for maintaining bone health and reducing hot flashes or other symptoms of menopause, a good stretching session will make you feel better in general. As women age, it becomes more and more important to incorporate stretching activities into weekly routines. It's a great way to unwind and release the stresses of the day while doing something good for your body, allowing for better sleep and less soreness the next day. One of the authors goes through a regular stretching routine with her husband in the evenings.

Flexibility and stretching activities can be overlooked when trying to schedule work, family life, social activities, and time for exercising. Although the importance of cardiorespiratory fitness and the need for muscular strength and endurance may be obvious, in the crunch of lunch-hour fitness or early morning workouts, time for an additional 20 minutes of stretching during the cool-down can seem unrealistic. If stretching is performed, it is often hurried, without targeting the major joints of the body, the muscles used, and potential stiff areas.

No matter what your age or fitness level, good flexibility makes life easier. Your level of flexibility can be improved with a regular stretching program. Stretching exercises can be done almost anywhere with equipment no more complex than a towel or an exercise mat. Even when your schedule is tight and there is little time to exercise, basic stretching helps reduce stress and keeps the muscles flexible.

Stretching, flexibility, and warming up are not interchangeable terms. Flexibility describes a joint's ability to move freely through its full range of motion. Stretching usually involves an exercise that moves the joint, ligaments, muscles, and tendons through their ordinary range of motion and slightly beyond. Frequently, individuals will stretch by using a selected set of exercises for specific joints and muscle groups. Warming up is a general activity, potentially including calisthenics and stretching, to increase body temperature. The purpose of a warm-up is to prepare the body for the intended physical activity; warming up for 10 to 20 minutes should gradually elevate the heart rate and body temperature, making you ready for safe participation in your workout.

Flexibility Defined

Range of motion describes the amount of movement possible at a particular joint. Flexibility is the ability to move a joint or group of joints without injury through the full range of motion (Holt, Holt, and Pellham 1996). Flexibility allows you to twist, bend, turn, reach, and lift during activities of daily living. It is what provides the natural grace and efficiency to basic movements as well as to athletic activities. Without it, motion becomes stiff, jerky, and awkward. Flexibility fosters healthy joints and muscles and promotes the freedom of motion, thereby improving the quality of your life.

The level of flexibility or range of motion you possess is unique to you and will change throughout your lifetime. Females generally have greater range of motion than males because of anatomical and hormonal differences and the type of activities in which they often participate (Corbin et al. 2002). However, the differences depend on the joint and the movement involved. For example, women tend to have more hip flexion than men, but men demonstrate more hip extension (Heyward 2002). Heredity, age, body composition, and injuries also affect how flexible you are and can become. The length of your arms, legs, and torso can significantly affect your ability to stretch and reach. As you age, the muscles, tendons, and joints lose elasticity, so stretching becomes important to maintain flexibility and reduce the potential for injury and stiffness that may otherwise occur. Body fat can decrease the range of joint movement because of the amount of fat tissue around the joint and muscles. Additionally, previous muscle injuries, arthritis, and heavy scarring can also reduce flexibility of the joints.

Flexibility Facts

The type of joint—the location where two or more bones meet—partially determines the range of motion. Movement at a hinge joint such as the knee is only forward and backward, whereas a ball-and-socket joint such as the hip allows motion in multiple directions. Joint capsules enclose the major joints of the body and are composed of connective tissue that strengthens and reinforces the joint area. Joints with more connective tissue around them have excellent flexibility.

The soft tissues—the muscles, tendons, ligaments, and skin in a given location—also determine the flexibility in a joint. Muscles are the important component in flexibility because they can be lengthened to facilitate the range of motion regularly used (Current issues in flexibility fitness 2000). The composition of muscle includes contractile muscle fibers intertwined with connective tissue. Two main types of connective tissue fibers are important to discuss: collagen and elastin. Within connective tissue, collagen is the white fiber that provides strength and support, while elastin is the supple and elastic yellow fiber. Because connective tissue envelops every muscle fiber, the muscles exhibit properties of both elastin and collagen. Although the muscle fibers are fairly stretchable, the elasticity of connective tissue is limited. When these limits are reached, connective tissue becomes brittle and may tear when overstretched. Therefore, stretching should be gentle and gradual; to prevent injury, avoid bouncing and jerking movements.

Flexibility, like the other components of fitness, can be increased or reduced. With age, the extensibility of muscles and other soft tissues diminishes. To avoid the vicious cycle of flexibility loss, doing less, and continually becoming stiffer, it is important to regain, maintain, or improve your physical fitness level and avoid sedentary behaviors. When tying shoes, zipping a back zipper, swinging a golf club, or watching for cars in traffic become difficult, it's clearly time to start a basic stretching program. Whatever your age, stretching programs can be an effective way to maintain or improve your flexibility.

Muscular strength can affect flexibility. Normally, muscles on opposite sides of the joints are about equal in size and power. When a muscle imbalance occurs because of inactivity, injury, or overtraining, the range of motion at the joint changes. Tightness and lack of flexibility may result. An example is poor posture caused by continually leaning the head and shoulders forward, resulting in tightened chest muscles and stretched muscles of the upper back. Your mother may have scolded you about your posture. Maybe she knew that good flexibility is important for good posture.

Although conclusive evidence for a direct link between good flexibility and reduced risk of future injuries is lacking, benefits have been documented with regard to coordination and ease of movement (ACSM 2001). As aging occurs, aches and pains, poor posture, and guarded movements can lead to limited activity and a decrease in the range of motion in the joints. Consistent stretching to maintain and improve your flexibility can also prevent joint aches and muscle pain from becoming debilitating. Moving joints in a full range of motion increases flexibility and contributes to overall fitness and health.

Flexibility is joint-specific and changeable. You can have very limber shoulders yet be very stiff in the hips or hamstrings (muscles located in the back of the legs). Or, one shoulder may be tighter than the other. If it is, then try to stretch the tighter joint a little more until the range of motion is similar (Blahnik 2004). Injuries also contribute to stiffness of the joints and muscles, so take care in any stretching activity involving a previously injured joint. Inactivity and a lack of stretching can decrease flexibility, so the old saying "Use it or lose it" certainly applies. Therefore, a regular stretching program that incorporates the major joints and muscles improves and maintains flexibility and the freedom to move as you choose.

Benefits of Flexibility

A sensible flexibility program provides many benefits because a wide range of muscular and skeletal problems is associated with a lack of flexibility. Good flexibility can decrease the potential of muscle injuries and back problems. Flexibility can improve circulation, posture, gait, mobility, and general appearance. Additionally, a regular stretching program can help reduce the effects of daily stress and tension on the body.

If you have not previously been active and now understand how much benefit you receive from cardiorespiratory and strength workouts in reducing your menopausal health risks, flexibility will aid in the safe continuation of these activities. If you tend to get a little stiff from some of your new workout routines, gentle stretching is the answer. If you wake up in the middle of the night with hot flashes and cannot go back to sleep, why not stretch? You're already sweating and warm, so use it to your advantage; stretch your shoulders, back, and legs, then continue your night's rest.

Gentle stretching generally relaxes the muscles and is frequently used to relieve muscle cramps. As a part of the cool-down, stretching can reduce muscle soreness and recovery time after exercising. It loosens and lengthens the exercised muscles and increases the blood flow and circulation.

About 12 to 24 hours after exercising or performing unaccustomed activities, the muscles used may feel sore and stiff. Microscopic tears in the muscle fibers cause this soreness, referred to as delayed onset muscle soreness (DOMS). For the first two days after overexertion, the soreness is at its worst, then it begins to decrease (Ross 1999). Warming up and stretching the muscles to be used prepares your body for activity. Stretching these same muscles after the activity also helps prevent or minimize DOMS.

Individuals with a full range of motion in their joints possess better balance and overall coordination. Flexibility can decrease with aging, and this is often noticed in a person's gait. If the hips and ankles are inflexible, the stride becomes shorter, and there is less natural bounce when walking, jogging, or dancing. As you age, balance and coordination can help you maintain your mobility and agility. There is always the possibility of injury from falls, but flexibility can make falls less likely because you may be able to recover your balance and prevent the fall.

Stretching Methods

Several types of stretching exercises exist: static stretches, ballistic stretches, and PNF (proprioceptive neuromuscular facilitation) stretches. These types of stretching activities range from simple to complex. Of the three, static stretching is the safest and the one we recommend. It is a gentle, slow stretch (lengthening) of the muscle(s), held for 10 to 30 seconds. Stretch to the point of discomfort, release slightly, and then hold the stretch. Do not stretch to the point of pain.

Static stretching can be performed with or without some type of external aid to help you stretch (Blahnik 2004). Assisted stretching uses your body weight, gravity, a towel, or even a golf club to help as you stretch your muscles. It's easy to use assisted stretching, but care must be taken to avoid overstretching when gravity or your body weight is involved. Unassisted stretching, or active stretching, occurs when you contract one muscle to stretch another muscle (e.g., stretching the calf muscles by flexing the muscles in the shin). Unassisted stretching also builds strength while improving your flexibility (Blahnik 2004).

Ballistic stretching occurs when the muscles are stretched as the body bounces, swings, or jerks in an abrupt movement. Examples of ballistic stretching include doing several bouncing squats or bending over suddenly to touch your toes by bouncing down. This sudden overstretching causes the stretch reflex (a protective contraction of the muscle) to occur and can result in tightness in subsequent activities or in torn muscles and tendons. Joints can also be damaged during ballistic stretching. Therefore, although used by some athletes, we do not recommend ballistic stretching as part of a general exercise program.

In PNF stretching, contraction and relaxation of the muscle forms the basis of the stretching technique. First, the muscle is contracted against a resistance, then relaxed and stretched. Although the PNF procedure is effective, there are disadvantages. It can cause muscle soreness, and it requires more time to complete than static stretches because of the contraction–relaxation phases. Additionally, PNF stretching typically requires a partner to assist in providing resistance for the muscle contraction, thereby increasing the possibility of poststretching stiffness or muscle injury caused by too much force or a lack of communication between the individuals.

Assessing Flexibility

Because flexibility is specific to each joint, no single test can measure the flexibility of the total body (ACSM 2000). Therefore, several simple tests are used to determine flexibility in the shoulders, lower back, hips, and legs. These tests can also measure progress or maintenance of flexibility as you continue a regular stretching program. Remember to warm up and stretch the muscles adequately before assessing your flexibility. Also, avoid any fast or bouncing movements during the tests.

The sit-and-reach test is the most commonly used test of general flexibility. It measures the flexibility in the lower back and hamstrings and is viewed as an important predictor of musculoskeletal health in women (CSEP 2003). A sit-and-reach box with premeasured inches and a sliding bar beyond the toe point is easy to use. If this type of box is unavailable, a yardstick and a piece of tape will also work (see the following sidebar for details). Check your score for the sit-and-reach test in table 5.1.

▷ *Sit-and-Reach Test*

Put the yardstick on the floor, and place a piece of tape horizontally across it at the 15-inch point. Sit on the floor with the beginning point of the yardstick in between the legs, with your heels on the edge of the 15-inch taped line. The heels should be spaced in a comfortable position about 8 to 10 inches apart. To perform this test, keep one hand directly on top of the other, and do not lead with one hand or the other. Slowly reach forward along the yardstick as far as possible (see figure 5.1). The legs should remain fully extended, and the breath should not be held during this test. Hold this position long enough for a partner to measure the distance you reach. Repeat a second time and record the farthest distance.

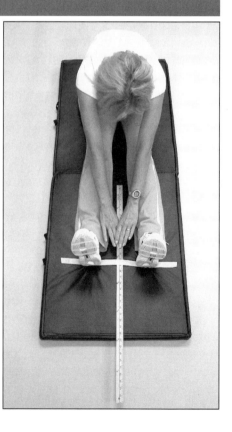

Figure 5.1 Sit-and-reach test position.

Table 5.1   Female Norms for the Sit-and-Reach Test (number of inches)

Rating	Age (years)		
	36-45	**46-55**	**56 and above**
Well above average	22 and above	21 and above	20 and above
Above average	19-21	18-20	17-19
Average	17-18	16-17	15-16
Below average	15-16	14-15	13-14
Well below average	14 or lower	13 or lower	12 or lower

Reprinted from *Y's Way to Physical Fitness, 4th edition,* with permission of the YMCA of the USA, 101 N. Wacker Drive, Chicago, IL 60606.

To assess the flexibility in the shoulders and upper arms, use the "zipper" stretch. (See figure 5.2 and refer to the description of this stretch later in the chapter.) A partner can assess your performance on this test. The fingertips should almost touch (ACSM 2001). Repeat with the arms in the opposite directions. Work to improve the range of motion in your shoulders if you find this stretch difficult. The ability to perform this and other stretches depends on a variety of personal factors. Some women may easily touch their fingertips on this stretch, while others struggle to get their arms and hands into position for this stretch.

The hamstring stretch assesses the range of motion for the muscles on the back of the thigh. Lie on your

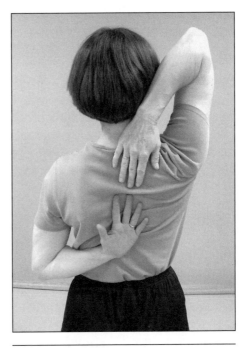

Figure 5.2   Zipper stretch.

back on the floor with knees slightly bent. To show good hamstring flexibility, you must lift one leg until it is nearly perpendicular to the floor while keeping the knee straight. The other foot should be resting on the floor (see figure 5.3). Repeat this test with the other leg. Have a partner compare your hamstring flexibility with the picture. Having tight hamstrings simply means you need to work on stretching these muscles in the future.

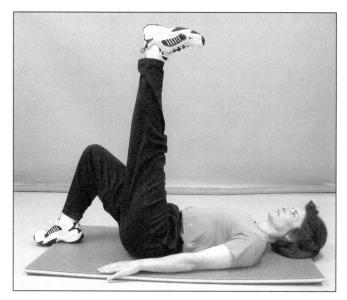

Figure 5.3 Hamstring stretch

Stretching Safely

Don't expect to simply jump into a great stretching session. Stretching is easier when the muscles are warm. If stretches are included as a part of the warm-up, it's best to first walk briskly with a good arm swing for about five minutes to increase muscle temperature (Knudson 1999). This warm-up of the muscles before stretching is especially important during cold weather (Ash and Werlinger 1997). During an exercise session, if you have only enough time to stretch once, then stretch after the workout as part of the cool-down.

Before stretching, the muscles should be relaxed and free of muscular tension. Gentle shaking of the limbs is helpful to loosen the muscles (Griffin 1998). You may have seen sprinters or swimmers loosening the muscles in their arms or legs before a race. Effective loosening exercises include leaning slightly forward and shaking the arm and hands, lying on your back with the knees bent and shaking the thigh and calf muscles, or lifting the shoulders in a shrugging motion and gently letting them fall (Griffin 1998).

Find a time when you can stretch for 20 to 30 minutes. Perhaps you can stretch during a TV show, to a relaxing CD, or as a part of an extended cool-down. The best results occur when you stretch every day, but two or three times a week is recommended as a minimum. All the muscle groups deserve a good stretch, but you should concentrate on the areas that generally lack flexibility or are most likely to become tight: neck, shoulders, chest, lower back, hips, thighs, and calves.

Remember to stretch slowly and gently and to avoid bouncing or jerky movements. Breathe normally while performing the stretches; don't hold your breath. Hold each stretch from 10 to 30 seconds, and repeat each stretch three or four times (ACSM 2001). Stretching should not hurt or be painful. You should feel mild tension in the muscle because you are moving the joint and muscle beyond its usual range.

Strained and injured muscles shouldn't be stretched, unless you are following the advice of a therapist or physician. If you have arthritis, stretch carefully and regularly. Consult your physician or physical therapist about stretching swollen joints. (See *Action Plan for Arthritis* by A. Lynn Millar [2003, Human Kinetics].) If you have osteoporosis, avoid stretching exercises that cause you to bend forward from the waist (Shangold and Sherman 1998). Seek the advice of your doctor regarding the best flexibility routine for your condition.

As you develop your own flexibility program, consider the following three concepts when you select and perform your stretches: variety, strength, and balance (Blahnik 2004). For variety, be sure to include both assisted and unassisted stretches as you work to increase your range in the tight areas. Unassisted stretches also allow for potential development of strength. Try to develop balance in your range of motion for nearly equal flexibility on the right and left sides of the body and on the front and back of the trunk, arms, and legs (Blahnik 2004).

Proper stretching is important to maintain or improve your flexibility. Stretching safely can reduce the possibility of unnecessary injuries. Some stretches are not recommended even though you might have previously performed some of these exercises. Avoid any stretch that puts excessive pressure or strain on a joint, ligaments, or the spine. Rolling the head in a complete circle can injure the neck. Standing and touching your toes can strain the lower back. The traditional hurdler's stretch shown in figure 5.4 can injure the ligaments of the knee. Full squats pose a triple threat to the knees, ankles, and spine. Lying on the back with the toes touching the floor behind the head poses a threat to the back, shoulders, and neck (see figure 5.5).

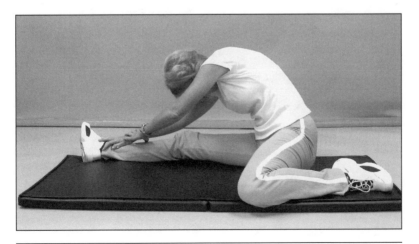

Figure 5.4 The traditional hurdler's stretch is not good for the knee ligaments.

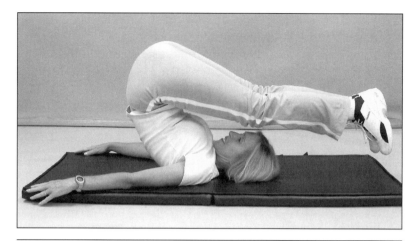

Figure 5.5 The plow position can injure the back, shoulders, or neck.

Safe alternatives are available for each of these unsafe stretches (see table 5.2). Head turns or head tilts stretch tight, sore, or achy neck muscles. Seated toe touches reduce the force of the stretch and strain on the back. Instead of a hurdler's stretch, modify it by rotating the bent knee and hip out, with the toes near the knee of the extended leg (see figure 5.6). This modified hurdler's stretch can be used as a safe substitute for full squats, along with a calf stretch. The neck, shoulders, and upper back can be stretched with individual stretches described later in this chapter.

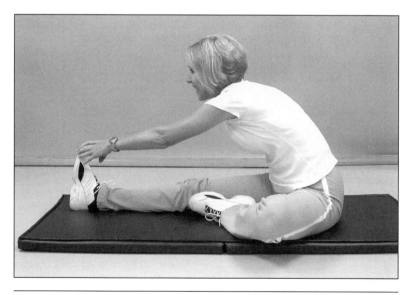

Figure 5.6 The modified hurdler's stretch is much safer than the traditional version.

Table 5.2   Alternatives to Unsafe Stretches

Unsafe stretch	Possible injury it causes	Safe alternative
Head circles	Injury to neck	Head turns or head tilts
Standing toe touches	Strains the lower back	Seated toe touches
Hurdler's stretch	Ligament injury to bent knee	Modified hurdler's stretch
Full squats	Knee, ankle, or spine injury	Modified hurdler's stretch and calf stretches
The plow (lying on back, touching toes on floor behind head)	Injury to neck, back, or spine	Individual stretches for neck, shoulders, and upper back

Developing Your Personal Stretching Program

Your flexibility program will also be determined by the activities and sports in which you most regularly participate. In addition to a comprehensive stretching program for the major muscle groups of the body, consider the muscles most involved in the activity and include specific stretches for them as well. For example, when cycling, the shoulders, neck, and legs need to be stretched before and during a long ride (Ash and Werlinger 1997). In racket sports, softball, and volleyball, the shoulders must be stretched with the knowledge that the dominant shoulder is the tighter shoulder because increased musculature on this side limits the range of motion (Griffin 1998). If you walk, jog, or run, the muscles in the legs need more attention in your routine. Golfers need to stretch the muscles in the back, hips, and shoulders.

Remember that simple stretches are not enough to protect you from all sports-related injuries. You need to possess adequate cardiorespiratory fitness and muscular strength and endurance, as well as flexibility, to participate in your chosen level of activities. If you are a beginner, take it easy and get your muscles, ligaments, and tendons accustomed to stretching and an increased range of motion.

Generally, it is better to stretch the muscles in the extremities and small joints before moving to the larger joints and muscles of the trunk (Corbin et al. 2002). For an organized flexibility routine, group together the stretches that require you to stand or lie down. To develop your personal flexibility routine, select the stretches you need for each major area of the body described in the next section. Table 5.3 provides the proper name of muscles or muscle groups discussed in the stretches. Write these in your stretching journal found in table 5.4 at the end of this chapter. (For more information on a wide variety of stretching routines, we recommend *Full-Body Flexibility* by Jay Blahnik [2004, Human Kinetics].)

Table 5.3 Muscles Found in Various Areas of the Body

Area of body	Name of muscles
Back of the neck and upper back	Trapezius
Front side of upper arm	Biceps
Back side of upper arm	Triceps
Shoulder	Deltoids
Chest	Pectorals
Back side of chest	Latissimus dorsi
Abdomen	Abdominals
Buttocks	Gluteals
Front of thigh	Quadriceps
Back of thigh	Hamstrings
Calf	Gastrocnemius and soleus
Inner thigh	Hip adductors
Outer thigh and buttocks	Hip abductors

HEAD TILTS AND HEAD TURNS

While looking straight ahead, move the right ear toward the right shoulder. Do not raise the shoulder. Repeat on the other side. A variation of this stretch is to turn the head to the right and hold, then turn to the left and repeat. These stretches release the muscle tension in the neck muscles and upper back.

ARMS ABOVE THE HEAD STRETCH

While sitting or standing, put your hands together and intertwine your fingers. Extend your arms and turn your palms away from the body. Raise your outstretched arms above your head. Reach as far up as possible. This stretch targets the triceps in the upper arms, as well as the upper back muscles.

Another arm stretch uses a rolled-up towel. Hold the towel in both hands behind the back. The thumbs should be facing out. Raise the towel as high behind the back as possible. This exercise loosens the shoulders, chest, and biceps muscles.

ZIPPER STRETCH

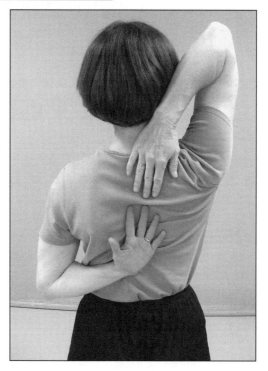

Lift one arm overhead, bend this elbow, and reach down the back toward the opposite shoulder. At the same time, bend the other arm behind the back with fingers up to touch the fingers of the opposite hand. A towel can be held in the upper hand to facilitate this stretch with a gentle pull from the lower hand. Repeat on the other side. The zipper stretch can be performed while standing or in a seated position. This exercise helps you reach your back zippers, and it stretches the triceps, front of the shoulder, and the back sides of the chest (latissimus dorsi).

HANGING STRETCH

Hang from a pull-up bar at the gym or the monkey bars at the playground. Depending on your strength and shoulder tightness, you may need to hang from a lower bar and keep some of your weight on your feet. This stretch improves the flexibility in your back and arm muscles and your lattissimus dorsi.

ARM ACROSS THE BODY STRETCH

Raise the right arm to shoulder height and reach across the body. With the left hand, grasp the right arm above the elbow and gently pull. This stretches the shoulder, and upper back. Repeat with the left arm.

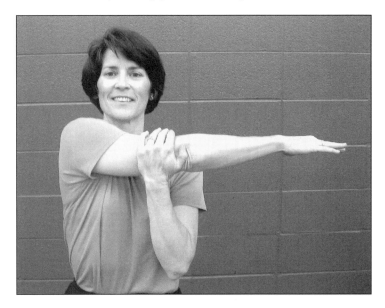

CHEST STRETCH

In a doorway, raise the arms almost to shoulder level, and bend the elbows to 90 degrees. Place the palms on the doorjambs, and gently lean forward through the doorway. Hold the stretch and repeat. This stretch can also be done in an empty corner by facing the corner and placing the arms against the walls at shoulder height. A third alternative for a shoulder stretch is to lace your fingers behind your head, with elbows out to the sides. Move your elbows back until you feel your chest muscles stretching. Hold and repeat to lengthen the chest (pectoral) and shoulder muscles.

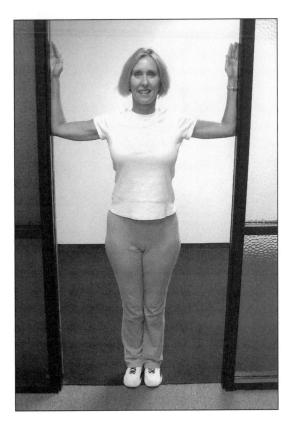

SIDE STRETCH

To stretch the muscles along the sides of the trunk, stand with your feet shoulder-width apart and knees slightly bent. Raise the left arm overhead, and place the right hand on the right hip. Slowly bend sideways to the right. You will feel the tension along the left side from the hip to the elbow. Repeat on the other side.

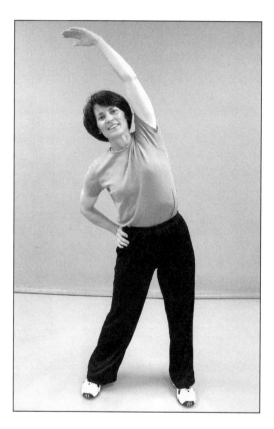

PRONE PRESS-UP STRETCH

Lie face down on the floor, with palms on the floor and the elbows bent. Keeping the forearms on the floor, gently raise the upper body until the elbows are at right angles (90 degrees) and directly under the shoulders. Keep the pelvis on the floor, and hold this position to stretch the abdominal muscles. Remember, there should be no pain when stretching.

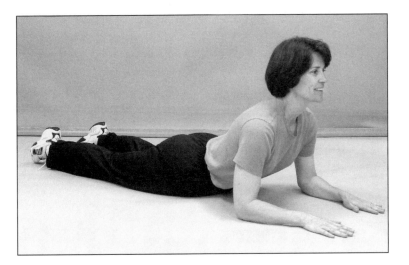

CAT BACK STRETCH

Kneel on the floor with your knees directly under your hips and your hands directly under the shoulders. Tighten the abdominal muscles and pull them up toward the backbone. Repeat this exercise to stretch the lower back muscles.

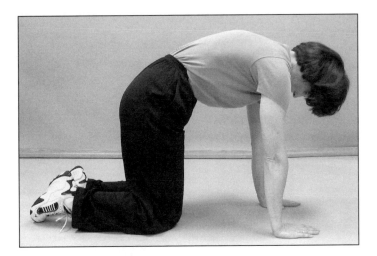

QUAD (UPPER THIGH) STRETCH

Stand and use the back of a chair or a wall for balance. While bending the right knee, raise the foot toward the buttocks. Reach behind your back with the left hand, and grasp the top of the right foot. Keep the thighs of both legs close together. Tighten your abdominal muscles, and gently pull the heel toward the buttocks. You should feel the stretch in the front of the thigh. Repeat on the left leg. This stretch reduces the tightness of the upper thigh that occurs from poor posture, sitting too long, or cycling and jogging.

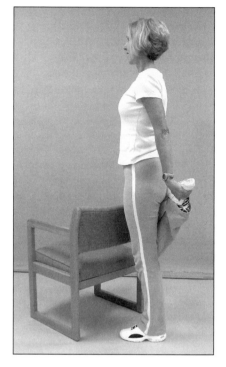

SIT-AND-REACH STRETCH

Sit on the floor with both legs together, straight and flat on the floor in front of you. Slowly lean forward, keeping the lower back flat, and reach ahead as far as you can. Repeat. (See the picture for the sit-and-reach test on page 118.) You may prefer to stretch your hamstrings one leg at a time. If so, sit in a modified hurdler's position, as shown in the photo: right leg straight and the right leg bent, with the sole of the left foot near the right knee. Keeping the lower back flat, reach the arms forward along the right leg as far as you can. Repeat on the other leg. Another variation of this stretch is to sit with the legs straight and comfortably spread apart. Stretch and hold on each side and also to the center. Perform these stretches to relieve tightness in the lower back, hamstrings, and buttocks (gluteal muscles).

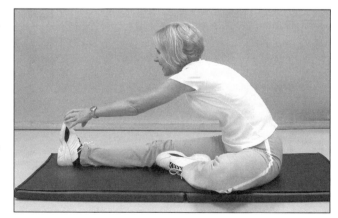

KNEES TO CHEST STRETCH

While lying on your back, pull both knees toward your chest. Grasp the back of your knees to stretch the muscles of the lower back and on the back of the thighs (hamstrings). This stretch could also be performed with one leg at a time by bending the leg of the knee not being pulled to the chest, keeping the foot flat on the floor.

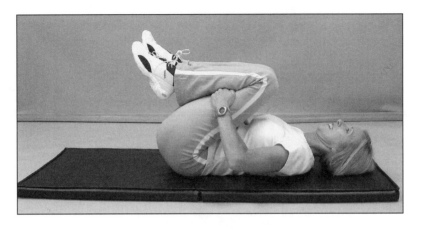

CALF STRETCH

Stand an arm's distance away from a wall with feet shoulder-width apart. Step one foot forward, and place both hands against the wall. Keep both feet flat on the floor, and bend the forward knee. Lean toward the wall, feeling the stretch in the calf muscle of the back leg. Repeat on the other leg. Calf stretches reduce stiffness in the lower legs caused by prolonged standing, wearing high heels, walking, and running.

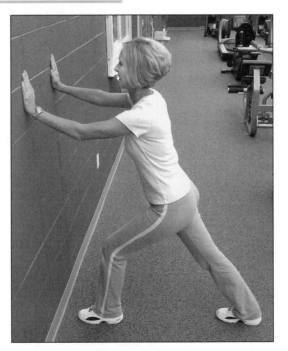

SIDE LUNGE STRETCH

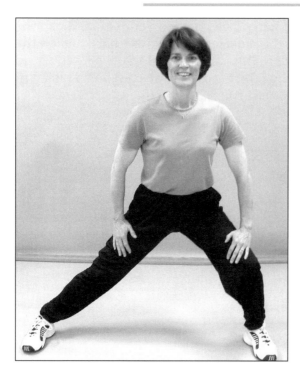

Stand with your feet wider than your shoulders, and place your hands on your thighs. Bend one knee and lower the hip until the other leg is straight. The weight should be over the bent knee in a side lunge position. Hold and stretch in the opposite direction to loosen the muscles on the inside of the thighs.

INNER THIGH STRETCH (BUTTERFLY STRETCH)

To reduce stiffness in the inner thigh muscles, sit with the knees bent and the soles of the feet as close as possible to the body. Lean forward

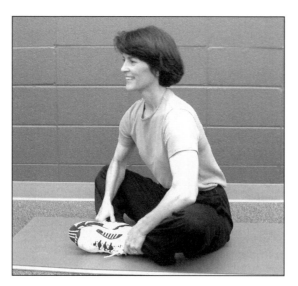

and press your forearms or elbows on the inner part of the thigh; press the legs outward toward the floor.

STANDING CROSSED LEG STRETCH

Stand and cross the right leg in front of the left leg, with the toes turned slightly out. Reach your right arm overhead and stretch overhead, leaning slightly to the left. Repeat on the other side. This exercise helps runners and those who have tightness and soreness in the outside of the knee or hip.

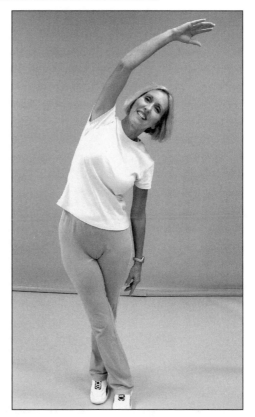

LUNGE STRETCH

Stand in a lunge or stride position, with the left leg two to three feet in front of the right. Bend the right knee until it touches the floor. The left knee should be directly above the left ankle. Place your hands on the back of your hips. Keep the lower back flat, and use your hands to push your hips forward and slightly up. You will feel the stretch in the front of the hips and quadriceps. Repeat with the other leg. This stretch decreases tightness that occurs in the upper thighs from prolonged sitting, walking, jogging, and cycling.

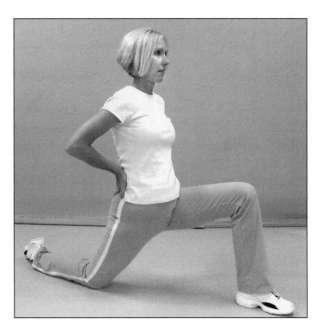

TRUNK TWISTER

Sit on the floor with the right leg extended in front of you. Bend the left knee, cross the left leg over the right, and put the left foot on the floor. Place the left hand on the floor behind the left hip. Turn the trunk to the left as far as possible, and push on the left thigh with the right arm. Stretch and hold this position. Repeat on the other side to stretch the trunk, outer thigh, hip muscles, and lower back.

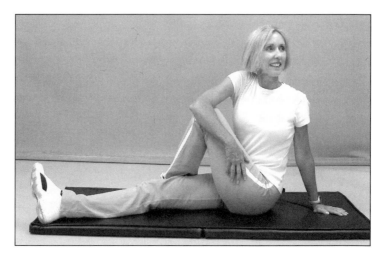

LYING BACK TWISTER

Lie on your back with both knees bent and your arms outstretched on the floor at shoulder height. Roll both hips and knees to the left, and gently turn your head to the right, feeling the stretch from the gluteals all the way to the upper arm. Stretch the other side.

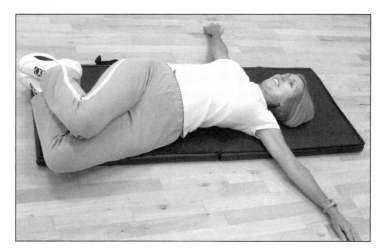

Frequency, Intensity, and Duration

According to the American College of Sports Medicine (2001), to maintain flexibility a person should stretch at least two or three days a week and preferably after moderate to vigorous physical activity. The amount of flexibility you require will be determined by your personal needs and fitness goals. Some women need to stretch only the minimum times per week; others need to stretch more often to achieve their desired goals. The more stretching you do, the more flexible you will become. Stretching daily or even several times a day can significantly increase your flexibility. Improvement in your flexibility usually occurs within four to five weeks (deVries 1981; Beaulieu 1980).

Each stretch should be slow and gentle. Stretch the muscle to the point of discomfort, and then release slightly. Hold this position for 10 to 30 seconds and breathe normally. Beginners should work to increase the range of motion in the major muscles and joints (hips, lower back, hamstrings, and shoulders). Stretch the opposite side, and repeat each stretch three or four times. Remember that flexibility is reversible, so plan to make stretching a part of your lifetime fitness and stress management routine.

Example of Sally's Flexibility Routine

Sally is learning how great she feels now that she has started a regular stretching routine. Because Sally is an elementary school teacher, she spends a great deal of time standing and walking during the day. Her legs are very tired, achy, and stiff by the end of a hectic day at school. Additionally, she knows that tension and stress build up in her neck, shoulders, and upper back. After work, Sally's usual routine is cardiorespiratory exercise on Mondays, Wednesdays, and Fridays. After her workout, she's ready to stretch. Her flexibility routine includes the following stretches: head tilts and turns, zipper stretch, arm across the body stretch, chest stretch, prone press-up stretch, calf stretch, quad stretch, knee to chest stretch, sit-and-reach stretch, standing crossed leg stretch, and trunk twister. After completing four of each of these stretches, Sally's ready for a shower, dinner, and some relaxing time.

Table 5.4   Weekly Stretching Journal

In addition to the stretches listed below, select additional stretches that will be most helpful to you. Each stretch should be slow and gentle. Stretch to the point of discomfort, release slightly, and then hold the stretch. Hold this position for 10 to 30 seconds and breathe normally. Stretch the opposite side, and repeat the stretch three or four times. Plan to stretch at least two or three times a week. Check the stretches that you perform during your stretching routine.

Type of stretch	Sunday	Monday	Tuesday	Wednesday	Thursday	Friday	Saturday
Head tilts and turns							
Zipper stretch							
Chest stretch							
Calf stretch							
Quad stretch							
Knee to chest stretch							
Sit-and-reach stretch							
Prone press-up stretch							

From *Action Plan for Menopause* by Barbara Bushman and Janice Clark Young, 2005, Champaign, IL: Human Kinetics.

Summary

Based on the information presented in the previous chapters, you know why exercise has the potential to help you move through menopause with less discomfort and side effects. After reading this chapter, take some time to consider your flexibility needs. What muscles are often tight or sore? What movements are becoming more difficult than they used to be? What activities do you want to continue or improve? Consider how a stretching routine can help you relax and not be stressed about the hormonal changes occurring at this time in your life. Your stretching plan should be unique to your body, its specific needs, and your present fitness goals. There is no one-size-fits-all flexibility routine. Analyze your schedule to find two to three times a week when you can stretch for about 20 minutes. Choose the exercises that are best for you, then start stretching to maintain or increase your range of motion and decrease your tension and stress.

ACTION PLAN:
STRETCHING AND LENGTHENING MUSCLES

☐ Stretch safely:
  • Warm up before stretching.
  • Stretch gently and hold for 10 to 30 seconds.
☐ Evaluate your present level of flexibility:
  • Select stretches to target areas needing improved flexibility.
  • Select stretches to maintain areas with good flexibility.
  • Periodically, perform the sit-and-reach test, shoulder flexibility test, and hamstring flexibility test to assess your progress.
☐ Select specific stretches that will complement your cardiorespiratory and strength workouts.

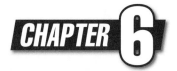
DESIGNING YOUR PERSONAL EXERCISE PROGRAM

The previous three chapters described the three legs of a complete exercise program: cardiorespiratory fitness, muscular fitness (strength and endurance), and flexibility. Each component is important and should be included in your exercise schedule. The options for your exercise program are truly limitless. This chapter includes some suggested plans for beginners as well as intermediate or established exercisers. We have included suggestions for traditional as well as nontraditional exercise. Your selection of exercise opportunities should reflect your current fitness and health status as well as your interests.

Aerobic Exercise

Your overall plan of action involves cardiorespiratory (aerobic) activity on three to five days, resistance training on two or three days, and stretching on two or three days. The American College of Sports Medicine has suggested a reasonable exercise progression for aerobic activity, which is outlined in table 6.1 (adapted from ACSM 2000). The levels are determined rather subjectively. Beginners are those women initiating an exercise program for the first time. The intermediate level includes approximately four to five months of progressive increases or improvements. The exact progression depends on your age and entry fitness level. Consider what your current fitness program includes, and begin

Table 6.1 Exercise Progression for Aerobic Activity

Your level	Number days per week	Exercise intensity		Time per session (or daily total)	Number of weeks at this work level
		RPE	% HRmax		
Beginner	3	11-12	50-55	15-20 min	1
	3-4	11-12	50-55	20-25 min	1
	3-4	12-13	55-65	20-25 min	1
	3-4	12-13	55-65	25-30 min	1
Intermediate	3-4	13-14	70	25-30 min	3
	3-4	13-14	70	30-35 min	3
	3-4	13-15	70-80	30-35 min	3
	3-5	13-15	70-80	30-35 min	3
	3-5	15-16	80-85	35-40 min	4
	3-5	15-16	80-85	35-40 min	4
Established	3-5	15-16	80-85	30-45 min	Onward!

Adapted, by permission, from American College of Sports Medicine (ACSM), 2000, *ACSM's guidelines for exercise testing and prescription,* 6th edition (Baltimore: Lippincott Williams & Wilkins), 154.

at that level. The maintenance level is the goal of three to five days per week of appropriate intensity exercise. For more information on determining exercise intensity using RPE or a percentage of your maximum heart rate, see chapter 3.

Progression within each fitness level depends on a number of factors including your age and baseline fitness. Beginner stage exercise may be too much if you have not previously been active at all. In that case, you should start with 5 minutes of easy activity (e.g., walking) a couple of times a day. Build up slowly by adding a minute or two to each session until you are able to exercise for 15 to 20 minutes continuously. At that point, you can begin at the first week on the chart.

For some of you, routine is the key. You may like to do basically the same activities each week. Some women enjoy walking at the mall or in their neighborhood without much variation in their aerobic workouts from week to week. Others enjoy a constantly changing series of activities. As long as you have the required fitness base, this can keep your workouts fresh and exciting.

As described in chapter 3, cardiorespiratory activities can be divided into different groups based on the skill level involved (ACSM 2000). We recommend that you begin with group one activities, which include activities you can easily maintain at a constant intensity and for which the caloric expenditure is similar between individuals. Walking is an example, and details on a walking program are given later in this chapter (other group one activities are listed in table 3.1 in chapter 3). Group two activities are more skill dependent and include activities in which, with the necessary skill, you can maintain a constant intensity, but the energy expenditure is relative to your skill level. An example from group two includes swimming because a certain skill level is required for a person to maintain the activity for a continuous period of time. We give some examples of swimming workouts that require good swimming skills, and thus those with a beginner fitness level may not be able to start immediately. Group three activities show wide variations in both skill and intensity and are most appropriate (and enjoyable) following the establishment of a fitness base through group one activities. Examples of group three activities include racket sports such as tennis and team sports such as soccer.

Walking

Walking is a simple activity with wonderful benefits, including improvements in cardiorespiratory fitness as well as a potential reduction in coronary heart disease (Manson et al. 1999). The simplicity of walking makes it appealing to many women. The equipment needed is minimal—good shoes. Purchasing quality walking shoes is recommended to allow you to enjoy your activity. When selecting a walking shoe, we recommend going to a reputable shoe store where your foot can be measured to ensure a good fit. Specifically look for a shoe with good shock absorption and arch support.

Walking location is a consideration—a track, sidewalk, or trail. Outdoor or indoor tracks are appealing because they provide an opportunity to record the distance completed. The surfaces also are more cushioned than if you were walking on a cement sidewalk. Initially, walking on a relatively level surface is recommended so the exertion level is constant and not too difficult. With increased fitness, tackling a hilly course might be appropriate to provide increased stress to the cardiorespiratory system. If you walk along a roadway, always face traffic and watch the approach of oncoming vehicles. For those with access, a treadmill also provides many options, with various speed and incline combinations.

In table 6.2, a sample walking plan is outlined. Note that various options are given for each of the fitness levels, reflecting progression in each stage. Some ways to add variety to your workouts (and also influence your RPE) include selecting a walking course with some changes in grade (i.e., hills) or using small hand weights (one to three pounds). When using hand weights, do not swing your arms excessively; rather, move your arms in a controlled fashion, focusing on good posture. Do not use ankle weights

Table 6.2   Sample Walking Program

Fitness level	Time point	Warm-up	Workout	Cool-down
Beginner	First week	Slow easy walking pace and gentle body stretches for 5 min	Walk at a pace that gives a fairly light level of exertion (RPE 11-12) for 10-15 min (3 days per week)	Slow easy walking pace for 5 min
	Later weeks	Slow easy walking pace and gentle body stretches for 10 min	Walk at a pace that gives a moderate level of exertion (RPE 12-13) for 20-25 min (3-4 days per week)	Slow easy walking pace for 10 min
Intermediate	Initial weeks	Slow easy walking pace and gentle body stretches for 10 min	Walk at a pace that feels somewhat hard (RPE 13-14) for 20-25 min (3-4 days per week)	Easy walking pace for 10 min
	Middle weeks	Slow easy walking pace and gentle body stretches for 10 min	Walk at a pace that feels somewhat hard to hard (RPE 13-15) for 25-30 min (3-5 days per week)	Easy walking pace for 10 min
	Later weeks	Slow easy walking pace and gentle body stretches for 10 min	Walk at a pace that feels hard (RPE 15-16) for 30-35 min (3-5 days per week)	Easy walking pace for 10 min
Established	Continue	Slow easy walking pace and gentle body stretches for 10 min	Walk at a pace that feels hard (RPE 15-16) for 30-40 min (3-5 days per week)	Easy walking pace for 10 min

when walking because they can interfere with your normal walking gait and cause potential injury to your joints.

Note that each week is not specifically outlined because each person will progress at her own rate. Slowly add time or intensity to your workouts (don't increase both at the same time). Your fitness program should involve a series of small changes rather than attempts at large increases in workload. A gradually progressive program will provide you with improvements in fitness while keeping muscle soreness to a minimum and the chance of injury low.

Swimming

Since swimming is a group two activity, we recommend starting a swimming program only after you have a fitness foundation (e.g., ability to walk for 30 minutes at a moderate level of exertion). Unlike walking, swimming requires more specialized skills. If you are familiar with the strokes, you will be able to make the transition into workouts relatively easily. If you do not have swimming skills, it is never too late to learn. Adult swim lessons are available at many community centers or through local universities.

Check the pool schedule of the local aquatic center for adult lap swimming times. At the pool, know the lap swimming rules for swimming with one or more people in your lane. Ask the lifeguard the procedure to follow if a swimmer in your lane needs to pass you. Select a lane with swimmers whose ability is similar to yours. For safety, swim only with a lifeguard on duty.

For fitness swimming, the best type of swimsuit is a cross-back tank suit (a one-piece nylon/Lycra suit with straps that cross in the back). Pool sandals will help avoid slips on wet pool decks. Swimming goggles and a silicone swim cap are needed to protect your eyes and hair. Always shower and wet your hair thoroughly before swimming in a pool. To keep your hair from absorbing so much chlorine, apply a small amount of conditioner to your wet hair and work it through your hair before putting on your swim cap. After your swim, use a shampoo that will remove chlorine from your hair, and use conditioner, too. After showering, to help your ear canals dry, put several drops of vinegar in your ears, then turn your head to let the solution drain out. The vinegar helps kill bacteria in the ear canal (Maglischo and Brennan 1985). One of the authors uses this economical alternative to the commercial preparations after every swim.

At most pools, pull buoys and kickboards are available for use. Pull buoys are pieces of shaped Styrofoam held between your legs to allow you to float while you work on your arm strokes. Kickboards (made from foam or Styrofoam) are held in your hands out in front of you and will help you improve your kicking ability. Both are indispensable as you complete your fitness swimming workouts. If your kick is initially weak, use a pair of swim fins to increase your ability and endurance. Pace clocks are the huge clocks on the pool deck or wall. Use the sweep second hand to check your pulse rate and to time your rest intervals when swimming.

In table 6.3, *pull* means to use a pull buoy and *kick* means to use a kickboard. Time intervals for rest are given as RI, so ":20 RI" means to rest 20 seconds before continuing. An asterisk (*) means you should check your heart rate for a 10-second interval. Note your heart rate as well as your RPE in your exercise log to be sure you are swimming at the proper intensity level. Heart rate tends to be lower in the water, so do not expect it to be the same as during on-land exercise. Using RPE is recommended in addition to taking your heart rate.

Table 6.3 Sample Swimming Program

Fitness level	Time point	Warm-up	Workout	Cool-down
Beginner	First week	Gentle shoulder and arm stretches, easy swimming pace for 5 min (change strokes as needed)	Use kickboard and swim laps (alternating strokes and type of kicking) at a fairly light level of exertion (RPE 11-12) for 10-15 min (3 days per week)	Easy swim pace (use favorite stroke) for 5 min, stretch calf and shoulder muscles
	Later weeks	Shoulder and arm stretches, easy pace swim and kick (change strokes and kicks as needed) for 10 min	Use kickboard, pull buoy, and swim laps (alternating strokes and type of kicking) at a moderate level of exertion (RPE 12-13) for 20-25 min (3-4 days per week)	Easy swim pace (use 2 favorite strokes) for 10 min, stretch calf and shoulder muscles Total distance: approximately 500 yd (depends on skill level)
Intermediate	Initial weeks	Shoulder and arm stretches, easy pace swim and kick (change strokes and kicks as needed) for 10 min	Use kickboard, pull buoy, and swim laps (alternating strokes and type of kicking) at a pace that feels somewhat hard (RPE 13-14) for 20-25 min (3-4 days per week)	Easy swim and pull for 10 min, stretch calf and shoulder muscles
	Middle weeks	Shoulder and arm stretches, easy pace swim and kick (change strokes and kicks as needed) for 10 min	Use kickboard, pull buoy, and swim laps (alternating strokes and type of kicking), keeping RI at :15-:20, at a pace that feels somewhat hard to hard (RPE 13-15) for 25-30 min (3-5 days per week)	Easy swim and pull for 10 min, stretch calf and shoulder muscles
	Later weeks	Shoulder and arm stretches, easy pace swim and kick (change strokes and kicks as needed) for 10 min	Use kickboard, pull buoy, and swim laps (alternating strokes and type of kicking), keeping RI at :10-:15, at a pace that feels hard (RPE 15-16) for 30-35 min (3-5 days per week)	Easy swim and pull for 10 min, stretch calf and shoulder muscles Total distance: 900-1,350 yd (depends on skill level)
Established	Continue	Shoulder and arm stretches, easy pace swim and kick (change strokes and kicks as needed) for 10 min	Swim, kick, pull, keeping RI at :10-:15, at a pace that feels hard (RPE 15-16) for 30-40 min; use repeated sets, ascending, descending, or Fartlek swims (3-5 days per week)	Easy swim and pull for 10 min, stretch calf and shoulder muscles Total distance: 1,500-2,000 yd (depends on skill level)

Note: For the workout, those with more advanced swimming skill can alternate strokes (freestyle, backstroke, breaststroke) and add repeated sets of swims, pulls, and kicks. For example: intermediate-skill swimmers: swim 2 × 50, 2 × 100 with RI of :15-:20; established swimmers: swim 4 × 100 with :10-:15 RI, kick 4 × 75 with :10-:15 RI, pull 6 × 50 with :10-:15 RI.

Cross Training in a Health Club

Health club memberships provide you with many, many options. Cross training simply means you use various activities rather than just one (e.g., a walking only program) to achieve your fitness goals. As you begin an exercise program, we recommend that you select group one activities and then add additional, more novel exercises as your fitness level improves. When trying new activities, keep in mind that you will likely be using your muscles in new ways, which may cause some soreness. Reduce your intensity and exercise time when learning a new skill. With class-type activities, don't let the momentum of the session pull you into doing more than you planned. Keep your focus on maintaining an appropriate RPE, and realize that learning the skills comes first and the intensity can be added later. In table 6.4 we give some options on how to add variety and progression to a cross training workout.

Table 6.4 Sample Cross Training Program at a Health Club

Fitness level	Time point	Warm-up	Workout	Cool-down
Beginner	Early weeks	Slow easy walking pace and gentle body stretches for 5 min	Pick one activity each day at RPE 11-12 (fairly light level of exertion) for 10-15 min (3-4 days per week): • Walking on the treadmill • Stationary bike	Slow easy walking pace for 5 min
	Later weeks	Slow easy walking pace and gentle body stretches for 10 min	Pick one activity each day at RPE 12-13 (moderate level of exertion) for 20-25 min (3-4 days per week): • Brisk walking on the treadmill • Stationary bike • Stair stepper	Slow easy walking pace for 10 min
Intermediate	Early weeks	Slow easy walking pace and gentle body stretches for 10 min	Pick one activity each day at RPE 13-14 (somewhat hard level of exertion) for 20-25 min (3-4 days per week): • Brisk walking or jogging on the treadmill • Stationary bike • Stair stepper • Elliptical trainer • Nordic ski machine	Easy walking pace for 10 min

(continued)

Table 6.4 *(continued)*

Fitness level	Time point	Warm-up	Workout	Cool-down
Intermediate *(continued)*	Middle weeks	Slow easy walking pace and gentle body stretches for 10 min	Pick one activity each day at RPE 13-15 (somewhat hard to hard level of exertion) for 25-30 min (3-5 days per week): • Brisk walking or jogging on the treadmill • Stationary bike • Stair stepper • Elliptical trainer • Nordic ski machine • Floor or step aerobics class	Easy walking pace for 10 min
	Later weeks	Slow easy walking pace and gentle body stretches for 10 min	Pick one activity each day at RPE 15-16 (hard level of exertion) for 30-35 min (3-5 days per week): • Brisk walking or jogging on the treadmill • Stationary bike • Elliptical trainer • Stair stepper • Nordic ski machine • Floor or step aerobics class • Spinning class	Easy walking pace for 10 min
Established	Continue	Slow easy walking pace and gentle body stretches for 10 min	Pick an exercise that provides you with an intensity that feels hard (15-16) for 30-40 min (3-5 days per week)	Easy walking pace for 10 min

Cross training is a great option for those who get bored with the same routine. Additionally, your body benefits from the unique training stimuli. Since the workload is not easy to determine for many of the activities listed, using your heart rate and RPE to monitor your exercise intensity is strongly recommended.

Other Group Two Activities

Group two activities are wonderful workout options for those possessing the required skill. Learning new activities can be fun and exciting. These activities would not be recommended for someone just starting an exercise program because the intensity may be too high—especially for those learning a skill, when efficiency is at its lowest.

Winter Activities

Do you enjoy crisp cold air on sunny winter days? Cross-country skiing on the local trails and golf courses (with permission, of course) is a great way to exercise and enjoy the beautiful winter scenery. The motion is nonjarring (at least as long as you stay upright!) and uses major muscle groups in the body. You can do cross-country skiing using the classical style (arms and legs move parallel and are synchronized, as with walking or running) or skating style (legs push in a lateral direction, similar to speedskating, with arms working to assist with the forward push). Selection of appropriate boots and skis is best made with the consultation of an experienced professional at a specialty shop. Shorter skis are more maneuverable, but longer skis are faster and smoother. You should select boots based on the terrain you plan to cover. Ski poles give a unique full-body workout because they assist in moving you forward in addition to keeping you upright. Different skiing styles require different-length poles, so consult an expert to fit you properly.

Ice skating is not just a winter sport if your community has a local ice rink. Check the open skating schedule at your community or university ice rink. Most have varied hours during the daytime, evenings, and weekends for open skating. If you are nervous about skating with crowds, watch for adults-only skating times. Enjoy the music while you skate. It helps make your skating more rhythmic and aerobic. If your skates are old, rent skates until you get back into skating form. Good skates make a huge difference in your comfort and ability to skate. Initially, work on basic stroking, stops, and inside and outside edges.

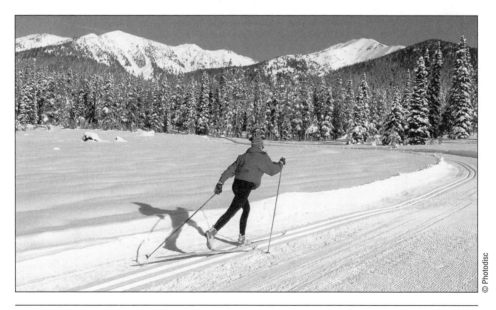

© Photodisc

Cross-country skiing is a great alternative to indoor aerobic exercise.

Summer Activities

Summer is viewed as time for sun, sand, and fun. Swimming and paddling are excellent ways to include some variety in your regular workout schedule. (Remember your sunscreen!) Enjoy yourself at the local pool or nearby lake. Act like a kid and splash, swim (above and underwater), and play. This much fun doesn't feel like exercise. You will be using muscles that you may not normally use, so move slowly into new activities.

While at the lake, rent a kayak. Once you have some instruction in proper paddling technique and water safety, you are ready for a great way to view the lake and get an excellent upper body workout. Be sure to wear a life jacket, and pay attention to the weather and water conditions, which could make a simple excursion turn into a potentially dangerous situation. Take along some water to keep well hydrated (for cool water all day, freeze a half-filled water bottle overnight, then top it off in the morning with cold water). When first sitting in the kayak, adjust the seat and foot pegs so you have some bend in your knees (to avoid strain on your lower back). Hold the paddle with hands approximately shoulder-width apart, keeping your hands relaxed—a tight grip is not necessary. When paddling, maintain good upper body posture. You want to stroke the water with a fluid motion that comes from your trunk rather than just your arms. Because kayak paddles have blades on each side, you will develop a rhythmic paddling motion as you become more experienced. Since you brace with your feet when kayaking, the leg workout is an added benefit.

Another fun summer activity is biking outdoors. Riding an appropriately sized bike will allow you to maximize your enjoyment; it may be worth going to your local bike shop to be fitted correctly. Adjust your seat so you have a slight bend in your knees at the bottom of the pedal stroke. Depending on the type of cycling you do, you may want to consider purchasing a pair of cycling shorts with a padded seat to increase comfort for longer bike rides. Many cities and towns have designated biking paths or even old railroads converted into walking and biking trails, which provide the benefit of no automobile traffic. When biking on roads open to automobiles, bike in the same direction as traffic, and adhere to all traffic rules (including use of hand signals when turning). Wearing bright clothing is a good way to increase your visibility to drivers. For safety always wear a properly fitted helmet. When it is hot, bike in the early mornings or evenings, and take some water along to maintain needed hydration.

Fitness Center Activities

The activity choices available at a fitness center may range from almost limitless to quite limited, depending on the center's facilities as well as its personnel and equipment. Most fitness centers typically offer classes in spinning and several types of aerobics. If a pool is available, deep water running and water aerobics may add enjoyable alternatives to your exercise program.

Deep water running. Deep water running involves going through the motions of running while in the deep end of a swimming pool. Your head is out of the water, with the waterline just above the shoulders. To maintain proper position, the use of a flotation device is recommended (various brands include Wet Vest, AquaJogger, and Thera-Band). The arms should be flexed at the elbows and move in a front-to-back motion, as when running on land. The forward motion should result in the fingertips coming almost to water level in the front; by the end of the backward motion, the fingers should be close to the hip. Keep the hands open to avoid cupping or pulling the water. The legs should move through a normal running stride. Since there is no contact with the ground, it is recommended that you dig your heel toward the bottom of the pool to simulate the foot hitting the ground. There is a tendency to either tread water (i.e., the hip does not go through the normal running range of motion) or keep the legs too far in front (i.e., sitting back in the water with legs moving in front of the trunk). The body should be positioned so the legs are under the torso, with a slight forward lean.

Since it is easy to become a human buoy, floating aimlessly around the pool, it is recommended that you take note of your rate of leg movement, or turnover. This is called your cadence. You may want to do constant intensity "runs" of 30 minutes at a moderate level of exertion. Another means to keep attention on your workout is to use intervals, or short periods of work interspersed with brief recovery periods. For example, a 30-minute workout could include the following:

Running for 4 minutes at a somewhat hard level of exertion, followed by 30 seconds of recovery

Running for 3 minutes at a somewhat hard level of exertion, followed by 30 seconds of recovery

Running for 2 minutes at a hard level of exertion, followed by 30 seconds of recovery

Running for 1 minute at a hard level of exertion, followed by 30 seconds of recovery

Running for 2 minutes at a hard level of exertion, followed by 30 seconds of recovery

Running for 1 minute at an easy level of exertion, then repeating the entire sequence

During the recovery periods, continue to move slowly through the water with a running motion as you allow your heart rate to slow down. To increase the intensity, increase your leg movement (turnover). Before and after any deep water running workout, you should include at least a 10-minute warm-up and 10-minute cool-down, including easy deep water running and gentle stretching activities.

Water aerobics. Water aerobics classes provide many workout options. Water depth (shallow to deep) is one consideration. Water is denser than air, and the movements of submerged body parts will meet with much greater resistance (thereby increasing the workload). Your level of comfort in the water may be one consideration when selecting shallow versus deep water aerobics. In a recent study of postmenopausal women, shallow water exercise allowed for maintenance of bone mineral density at the hip in addition to improvements in cardiorespiratory fitness, leg power, and flexibility over a 12-month period (Littrell and Snow 2004).

For water aerobics and shallow water walking or jogging, purchase a comfortable pair of water shoes for traction and to avoid abrading your feet on the pool floor. In addition to water shoes, various pieces of equipment are often utilized. The equipment used in water aerobics falls into four categories (Sanders 2000):

1. Buoyancy: flotation belts, kickboards, handheld flotation devices

2. Surface area: webbed gloves, paddles, swim fins

3. Integrated land/water: resistance bands or steps

4. Gravity: steps

This equipment uses your buoyancy and the water's resistance to provide an optimal workload.

The flow of a water aerobics session is no different from other workouts. A warm-up leads to the focused workout, followed by a gradual cool-down. The warm-up could include shallow water jogging in place as well as lateral and front-to-back movements. Gentle stretching can also be performed at the side of the pool. The main portion of the workout should focus on using large muscle groups in continuous, rhythmic movements (Sanders 2000). You can travel through the water or jog in place while in shallow water. When in deep water, bicycling motions with your legs, scissors kicks, and jogging in place are typical exercises. Cool-down activities should mimic the warm-up activities.

In addition to cardiorespiratory training, water aerobics also provide muscular strength and endurance training. You can use buoyancy, speed of movement, surface area, and inertia effects of the water to provide resistance (Sanders 2000). Focus on the work done by specific muscle groups, and adjust the speed of the movement (higher speed offers greater resistance in the water), or use a device to increase resistance (e.g., a webbed glove).

Flexibility exercises can also be incorporated for the upper and lower body. Moving joints through their range of motion may feel easier in the water because of the added support. In pools with cool temperatures, you may want to alternate some light jogging or movements with the stretching activities to keep warm (Sanders 2000).

Aerobics classes. Aerobics are a popular offering at most fitness facilities because of the variety of classes—all set to music. They include floor aerobics and step (bench) aerobics. Like any other well-designed workout, aerobics will incorporate a warm-up, main workout, and cool-down led by an instructor (who may always have her back to you). Classes are usually taught in rooms that have floor-to-ceiling mirrors so you can see the instructor (both front and back) to help you follow the step patterns. Classes range from beginner to advanced levels.

Shoes with adequate support and cushioning are a must for all aerobics-type classes. A quality fitness shoe is recommended (rather than a running shoe) to avoid turning an ankle when moving to the beat or stepping on and off the benches. Comfortable shorts and a shirt that allow free movement are also important.

If you have never taken any type of aerobics class (even if you are already in good cardiorespiratory condition), start with a beginning class to learn the basic steps and movement patterns. Grapevines, kicks, taps, turns, and straddle steps will soon become routine. (For step aerobics, absolute novices can view basic step patterns on the Internet by using "step aerobics" as the key search words.) In bench step aerobics, beginners usually start with the lowest step (four to six inches) and make incremental increases in the bench height as they progress. Regular monitoring of exercise heart rates or RPE will also occur during class. In all aerobics-type classes, have fun but stay within your heart rate intensity level when performing bench aerobics and using hand weights.

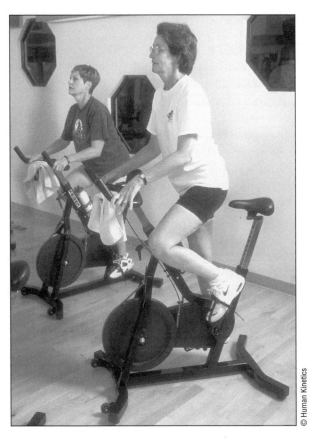

© Human Kinetics

Spinning classes. Spinning classes are offered at many health clubs and basically involve group stationary biking. A spinning class is led by a fitness instructor, often

Indoor cycling classes offer camaraderie with others in the class as you enhance aerobic conditioning.

to music, and should include a warm-up, workout phase, and cool-down. Before beginning the class, you should receive instruction on how to adjust your seat height and handlebar position, in addition to how the resistance is changed. Each brand of stationary bike is different, so do not hesitate to ask for assistance. You are able to adjust your workout (including resistance on the flywheel as well as your rate of pedaling) to match your current fitness level. The enthusiasm of the instructor can sometimes pull participants beyond their fitness levels, so be sure to monitor your RPE and make your own adjustments to the workload. The benefits of spinning classes include group camaraderie and a novel approach to a traditional activity.

Other Group Three Activities

In group three activities, skill and intensity can vary considerably. This can make monitoring intensity difficult, so listen to your body. Keep your overall perception of effort in mind (with RPE), and be willing to take breaks as needed.

Dancing

Most people who enjoy dancing usually don't view it as exercise. Whether you are dancing at a formal dance; sweating at a swing dance; line dancing; or practicing a jazz, tap, or clogging routine you are expending energy in a fun and social way. Whatever the dance type, dancing is a great way to get several hours of physical activity during weekly lessons or an evening out on the town.

When you dance, your energy expenditure is equivalent to walking one or more miles. Additionally, women benefit by increasing their shoulder and upper arm strength from holding their arms in dance position during that time. Good posture and proper alignment are important when dancing, so there is reinforcement in these areas, too.

If you are a baby boomer, then you probably never learned to dance with a partner. You can learn swing, Latin, or ballroom dance at community recreation centers or through local college and adult education courses. Group lessons will be the most economical, and you will meet many others at your ability level. Some local dance clubs also offer group dance lessons. If you are passionate about learning to dance, take private lessons with your partner. Dance instruction videos are also a good way to reinforce your skills.

The faster dances (cha-cha, salsa, swing, and hustle) use more energy than waltzes and foxtrots because of their faster foot patterns. As your dance skill improves, the calories burned while you dance and the length of time you can dance will increase (along with your enjoyment). Practice at home and rehearse in your living room. Then, go to a dance or a social situation where dancing occurs. The best way to improve your dancing is to regularly spend time on the dance floor.

Organized Leagues

Leagues are a great way to spend time with friends while exercising. A wide variety of options are available, including the following sports:

- Bowling
- Golf
- Tennis
- Racquetball and other court sports
- Volleyball
- Softball
- Soccer

This list has great variation in the amount of aerobic expenditure each activity provides. Pick one or more activities that you enjoy, and participate regularly. Don't try to be supercompetitive; just do your best as a team player and enjoy the camaraderie. These activities are much healthier for you (physically and socially) than sitting at home every night watching television.

Resistance Training

Resistance training plays an important part in your overall fitness program, allowing you to develop muscular strength and endurance. Using machines available at health clubs is a great option, but you can also do strengthening activities at home with minimal equipment. You should do resistance training two or three days per week.

Resistance Training at Home

For the following examples, you will need a resistance band and a set of dumbbells. Start with 5 to 10 minutes of walking and light calisthenics as your warm-up. For a beginner, the weight should be very light. It is important to perform the lifting movement correctly (to train the proper neuromuscular pathway in the muscles), as well as to exhale during the lift. Once familiar with the correct movement, select a weight that you can lift for at least 8 to 10 repetitions of the selected exercise. When you reach 12 repetitions in two consecutive workouts, increase the weight (Westcott and Baechle 1998). Select at least six to eight strength exercises for the legs, upper body, back, and abdominals. Those with more strength training experience typically include a second or third set of repetitions in their workout routines. Table 6.5 includes an example of an at-home strength workout. (You select the weight, number of repetitions, and number of sets.)

Table 6.5   At-Home Strength Workout

Body part	Exercise	Equipment needed	Amount of weight or band color	Number of repetitions	Number of sets
Legs	Wall squat	Wall			
Legs	Hip abduction	Resistance band			
Calves	Heel raise	Dumbbells			
Chest	Push-up, wall push-up, or modified push-up	Wall or none			
Chest	Upright row	Dumbbells or resistance band			
Shoulders and arms	Bench press	Dumbbells or resistance band			
Arms	Biceps curl	Dumbbells or resistance band			
Arms	Triceps extension	Dumbbells or resistance band			
Abdominals	Curl-up	Mat			

From *Action Plan for Menopause* by Barbara Bushman and Janice Clark Young, 2005, Champaign, IL: Human Kinetics.

Finish the workout with 5 to 10 minutes of walking and simple stretches for your arms and legs. (For more information on the specific exercises listed, see chapter 4.)

Resistance Training at a Fitness Facility or Gym

Resistance training at a fitness facility can provide you with additional options beyond what a home program can provide. Table 6.6 gives an example of a machine training workout. (You select the weight, number of repetitions, and number of sets.) Be sure to include a warm-up and cool-down. The goal is to incorporate two or three days per week of resistance training in your exercise program.

Table 6.6 Strength Training Program With Machines

Body part	Exercise	Amount of weight	Number of repetitions	Number of sets
Legs	Leg press			
Chest	Chest press			
Upper back	Compound row			
Arms and back	Lat pull-down			
Arms and back	Pull-up			
Arms and back	Chin-up			
Arms	Biceps curl			
Arms	Triceps curl			
Back	Back extension			
Legs	Hip abduction			
Legs	Hip adduction			
Abdominals	Abdominal curl			

From *Action Plan for Menopause* by Barbara Bushman and Janice Clark Young, 2005, Champaign, IL: Human Kinetics.

Flexibility

Details on a complete stretching program were given in chapter 5; however, you can stretch almost anywhere at almost anytime. Need a zero-calorie energizer at work? Perform head tilts or turns and the arm-across-the-body stretch, chest stretch, and calf stretch. Stuck in traffic? Do zipper stretches. Waiting in line at the grocery store? Try a standing crossed-leg stretch or a quad stretch while holding onto the shopping cart. Stretch while watching television, or carefully perform a sit-and-reach stretch while in the warm water of a bathtub or spa. You can stretch anytime your body is warmed up. Stretching at night is the perfect way to relax and release the day's stresses and tension from your muscles.

Summary

Our intent with this chapter is to demonstrate the many options for your exercise program. Each person has her own preferences and abilities. We (the authors) each rely on favorite activities as the mainstays of our personal workouts but include seasonal favorites for variety. At times the routine of consistently applied activities is enough (and may actually be a comforting constant as other life situations change). Trying new activities after you have established your fitness base can also add spice into an exercise program and can spark renewed enthusiasm.

ACTION PLAN:
DESIGNING YOUR PERSONAL EXERCISE PROGRAM

- ☐ Decide what activities are appealing to you and will allow you to focus on cardiorespiratory fitness, muscular fitness, and flexibility.
- ☐ Determine your progression over the upcoming weeks.
- ☐ Consider what alternative activities you might be interested in learning.
- ☐ Check into exercise or dance classes available in your community.
- ☐ Use the sample programs as a reference point to develop your own personalized exercise program.

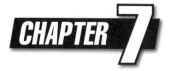

CHAPTER 7

BALANCING EXERCISE, NUTRITION, AND STRESS

Menopause is a continuation of the many transitions that have occurred since your conception and birth. Although previously menopause might have been mistakenly viewed as a woman's disease, it certainly is not a disease. Menopause is part of the natural course of living and aging among women.

It has been said that there are three stages to a woman's life: the maiden years, the mother years, and the crone years. The maiden years and the mother years have been and continue to be elevated or honored in most societies. Previously in some cultures, menopause was marked by ceremony as an entrance to the crone years. This celebration of the crone years as a time to utilize a woman's wisdom and life experiences has been lost with the current emphasis on youth. Rather than view menopause as a negative time of life, you should embrace each stage of life and live with vigor, zest, and a joy of living.

With many aspects of human development, adjustments must take place as you become accustomed to life changes. Although initially, you may not have enjoyed the changes menstruation caused in your life, its onset was marked with the knowledge that you had the ability to create life; you began to understand those opportunities and responsibilities during your reproductive years. Menopause requires other adjustments in daily living as the production of ovarian hormones decreases and finally ends. This chapter includes a discussion of the need for attaining proper nutrition, handling stress, and reducing the potential of disease as you live the rest of your life in the menopausal years. It also provides information on maintaining your sexual health and recommendations for continued health examinations and tests.

Striving for Proper Nutrition

If you have not given much attention to your personal nutrition, now is the time to start. Maybe you have been too busy helping others—children, spouse, family, and friends—but it is critical for you to pay close attention to your nutritional needs at this point in your life. Calories are part of the equation, but more important you need to eat foods that provide adequate nutrients for your body's changing needs.

If the idea of a healthy diet sounds like a dreary sentence from a strict dietitian, then it's time for a change to a positive perspective. Women need to eat to live, not live to eat. Even though you would never dream of putting a mixture of Kool-Aid, orange juice, and water in your automobile gas tank, you might ingest any mixture of caffeine, sugars, salt, fats, empty calories, and prescription or over-the-counter drugs and think you are fueled for the day. Unlike a car engine, your body will run on just about any fuel, although long-term repercussions may result. This section discusses the function of nutrients and how to plan for a high-octane daily menu.

Six Essential Nutrients

There are six essential nutrients. Of these, three (carbohydrates, fats, and proteins) supply calories and produce energy for the body. Carbohydrates and proteins supply four calories per gram, while fats provide nine calories per gram. The other three essential nutrients are water, vitamins, and minerals. They do not provide calories for energy but assist in the body's growth, structural, and regulatory processes as well as the release of energy from foods (Williams 2002). A balanced daily diet should contain 45 to 65 percent carbohydrates, 10 to 35 percent protein, and 20 to 35 percent fat (Directory Guidelines for Americans [DGA] 2005a).

Carbohydrates

Carbohydrates have the primary function of supplying the body with energy; they are the preferred source of energy for the brain and nervous system (Wardlaw 2003). There are two types of carbohydrates: complex and simple. Simple carbohydrates are the sugars found naturally in fruits, some vegetables, and milk, as well as the sugars found in honey, syrups, and the sugar bowl. The simple carbohydrates found in desserts and candies are often accompanied by fats; therefore, you should limit your intake of these in your daily diet.

Complex carbohydrates consist of starches and fiber and include whole grains, cereals, pastas, fruits, and vegetables. These complex carbohydrates should be the foundation of your diet, making up the majority of the 45 to 65 percent daily carbohydrate intake. A diet high in complex carbohydrates is often rich in vitamins and minerals and low in saturated fats, thereby potentially reducing the risk of diabetes and cardiovascular diseases in women (American Dietetic Association [ADA] 2004).

Dietary fiber (aka roughage) is found only in plant foods. Humans are unable to digest these plant fibers. There are two forms of fiber, soluble and insoluble, and both can aid in weight control since they prolong chewing time and make the stomach feel full longer because they absorb water (ADA 2002a). Insoluble fibers (wheat and corn bran, leafy vegetables, and skins of fruits and root vegetables) increase fecal bulk and prevent constipation. Eating adequate amounts of fiber is part of the dietary plan for the treatment of cardiovascular diseases, diabetes, and diverticulitis and is associated with a lower risk of colon cancer (ADA 2002a). Soluble fiber (found in beans, barley, oats, and pulp of fruits and vegetables) lowers blood cholesterol and improves the body's ability to control blood sugar levels (ADA 2002a). The current recommendation for daily fiber intake is 20 to 35 grams of fiber a day (ADA 2002a), or to base the amount on your caloric consumption, 14 grams of fiber per 1,000 calories consumed in your diet (DGA 2005b).

Fat

Fat provides a concentrated source of energy from foods (at nine calories per gram, fats supply 2.5 times that of carbohydrate or protein). It can be stored in basically unlimited amounts by the body as a future energy reserve. Fats play important roles within the body, including serving as carriers for fat-soluble vitamins, components of all cell membranes, and sources of antioxidants. Fats are termed either saturated or unsaturated (in reference to their basic chemical structure). Saturated fats include animal fats, dairy fats, and tropical fats (coconut, palm, and palm kernel oils) (Singh 2000) and are usually solid or semisolid at room temperature, while unsaturated fats are less firm and more liquid. Extra dietary saturated fat contributes to increased blood levels of total cholesterol and low-density lipoprotein (LDL) cholesterol (which is often termed "bad" cholesterol) (American Heart Association [AHA] 2004a). Your daily intake of saturated fats should be below 10 percent of energy intake (DGA 2005a) and below 7 percent if your LDL cholesterol is high (more than 130 mg/dL). Trans fatty acids found in margarines and shortenings used in processed, baked, and fried foods have the same effect on the body as saturated fats (Singh 2000) and should be kept as low as possible, 1 percent of energy intake or lower (DGA 2005b). When your consumption of dietary fat is excessive, there is an increased risk of atherosclerosis, cardiovascular disease, and obesity, as well as breast cancer (AHA 2004a).

Unsaturated fat can be divided into monounsaturated and polyunsaturated, again based on chemical structure. Unsaturated fats are plant fats. Monounsaturated fats include canola, olive, and peanut oils. These fats are the preferred type of fat because of their potential benefits on HDL cholesterol ("good" cholesterol) and blood clotting (Williams 2002); the recommended daily amount of monounsaturated fats is up to 15 to 20 percent of daily calories (ACSM 2001; DGA 2005b). Polyunsaturated fats include soybean, corn, sunflower, and safflower oils. Although beneficial in reducing total cholesterol and LDL levels, polyunsaturated fats may also reduce HDL cholesterol as well as play a role in the development of colon cancer; therefore, you should limit your dietary intake of polyunsaturated fats to approximately 10 percent of your daily calories (Williams 2002).

Protein

Protein is a vital component of a healthy diet and should make up 10 to 35 percent of your daily caloric intake. Without protein, no new living tissue could be formed (Boyle and Zyla 1996). Complete proteins are found in meat, fish, and dairy products. Incomplete proteins are found in plant sources, although combining various plant sources can provide complete protein. For example, combining grains and legumes within a 24-hour period allows the body to utilize the various component parts to produce proteins that are equivalent to the complete proteins found in meat and fish. Peanut butter on 100 percent whole wheat bread is an example of combining plant-based foods to create complementary proteins. Eating beans and corn or tofu and rice are other examples.

Despite the current popularity of high-protein diets, there are no known benefits from excessive consumption of foods high in animal protein. Typically, diets high in animal protein are high in calories and saturated fat. As a result, these diets can potentially lead to increases in cholesterol levels, obesity, and the associated risks of coronary heart disease and cancer (Wardlaw 2003). Additionally, high-protein diets can cause increased calcium excretion, which can reduce bone density (Williams 2002) and initiate osteoporosis.

Vitamins, Minerals, and Water

The last three essential nutrients are vitamins, minerals, and water. These nutrients supply no energy or calories to the diet but do help release energy from the foods you eat. Water is needed in large amounts each day for good health, especially when exercising or during humid conditions.

Vitamins are required in very small amounts (milligrams and micrograms) and have a variety of distinct functions. They help release energy from carbohydrates, aid in the metabolism of fats and proteins, assist in growth and repair of tissue, facilitate bone and tooth formation, stabilize cell membranes, and assist in blood clot formation (Williams 2002; Wardlaw 2003). Vitamins are found in plentiful quantities in fruits, vegetables, and grains. Additionally, some foods are vitamin fortified, such as cereals and milk. Table 7.1 provides good sources of vitamins from each of the food groups.

Table 7.1 Sources of Vitamins in Foods

Food group	Vitamins found	Good sources
Grain group	Niacin	Brown rice, whole wheat bread, oatmeal
	Riboflavin	Whole wheat bread
	Thiamin	Whole wheat bread, brown rice
Vegetable group	Vitamin A	Sweet potato, carrot, spinach, butternut squash, turnip greens
	Vitamin C	Broccoli, brussels sprouts, cauliflower, baked potato, tomato
	Vitamin K	Turnip greens, spinach, cabbage, cauliflower, broccoli
	Riboflavin	Spinach, asparagus, broccoli
	Folate	Asparagus, spinach, black-eyed peas, romaine lettuce
Fruit group	Vitamin A	Cantaloupe, mango, dried apricots, papaya
	Vitamin C	Papaya, cantaloupe, orange, grapefruit, strawberries
	Folate	Cantaloupe, orange, strawberries
Milk group	Riboflavin	Nonfat milk, cottage cheese, ricotta cheese, cheddar cheese
	Vitamin A	Beef liver, flounder
	Vitamin D	Nonfat milk
	Vitamin B-12	Cottage cheese, plain yogurt, nonfat milk, cheddar cheese
Meat and beans group	Vitamin B-6	Pork, beef, tuna, chicken, soybeans, navy beans
	Vitamin B-12	Chicken liver, sardines, tuna, ground beef, shrimp, egg
	Niacin	Chicken breast, tuna, peanuts, fish, beef, pork, kidney beans
	Thiamin	Ham, pork, sirloin steak
	Vitamin D	Shrimp
Oils	Vitamin A	Margarine, butter
	Vitamin E	Safflower, canola, corn, olive, peanut, and sesame oils

Data from M.A. Boyle and G. Zyla, 1996.

Minerals facilitate muscle contractions and nerve transmission, aid in regulating metabolism, assist in energy utilization, and build bones and teeth (Williams 2002). Table 7.2 provides good sources of minerals from all the food groups. Deficiencies and excesses of either minerals or vitamins can create adverse health conditions.

Although you could survive for days and months without vitamins and minerals, you can quickly dehydrate and die without water, making it the most essential nutrient. Every cell, organ, and tissue of the body contains water. It is found in nearly all foods but especially in fruits and vegetables. Water is lost every day through sweat, urine, feces, and the act of breathing.

It is important that you maintain an adequate fluid intake. The average adult female needs about two quarts (eight cups) of water a day (Williams 2002), with more needed for exercise and during hot, humid weather. Do not rely on your thirst as a guide to the amount of fluids needed. By the time you are thirsty, you are already partially dehydrated. Drink water on a regular schedule—before you are thirsty. The more active you are, the more fluids you need: Drink at least one glass of water before and after exercising and a glass of water every 10 to 15 minutes during exercise (ACSM 2003a). If you are a caffeine fan, do not substitute coffee, tea, or sodas for water. More important, avoid alcoholic drinks to prevent dehydration. Signs of mild dehydration include dry mouth, lethargy, headache, and reduced urine output or very yellow urine (Singh 2000).

Nutrient Density

As you age, your metabolism slows, and a steady weight gain can occur during perimenopause and postmenopause if you continue to eat the same amount of calories. You can combat this by sensible and wise nutritional choices. A nutrient-dense food is one that contains the most nutrients with the least amount of calories (Williams 2002). For example, one cup of skim milk with its 86 calories is more nutrient dense than 2 percent milk containing 121 calories or whole milk containing 149 calories (Wardlaw 2003). Nutrient density is another good reason to read food labels, compare similar food products, and make wise food choices.

Making Wise Choices

The American College of Sports Medicine provides several important guidelines to follow in their Active Aging Partnership and the Strategic Health Initiative on Aging (ACSM 2003b). These guidelines include "Five Ways to Eat Better" and "Five Reasons to Eat Well," which are included in the sidebar on pages 164 and 165.

Table 7.2   Sources of Minerals in Foods

Food group	Minerals found	Good sources
Grain group	Iron	Bran cereal with raisins, oatmeal, whole wheat bread
	Zinc	Bran cereal with raisins, whole wheat bread
	Magnesium	Bran cereal with raisins
Vegetable group	Iron	Baked potato, lima beans, black-eyed peas, Swiss chard, spinach
	Magnesium	Spinach, baked potato, lima beans
	Potassium	Baked potato, lima beans, spinach, bok choy, tomato, broccoli
	Calcium	Collard and turnip greens, bok choy, broccoli
Fruit group	Potassium	Banana, orange juice, cantaloupe, raisins
	Iron	Prune juice, dried figs, dried apricots, raisins
Milk group	Calcium	Low-fat yogurt, cheese, nonfat milk, pudding, ice milk
	Phosphorus	Cheese, yogurt, nonfat milk
	Potassium	Nonfat milk
Meat and beans group	Iron	Clams, beef liver, beef, shrimp, sardines, navy beans, tuna
	Phosphorus	Salmon (canned), pork, beef, turkey, peanuts, navy beans, tuna
	Calcium	Sardines with bones, shrimp, salmon with bones, almonds, beans
	Potassium	Pork, hamburger, chicken
	Magnesium	Almonds, cashews, hamburger, pork
	Zinc	Oysters, sirloin steak, beef, crabmeat, turkey, peanuts

Data from M.A. Boyle and G. Zyla, 1996.

Almost all nutrition guidelines and recommendations advocate that the majority of the American diet should include more plant-based whole foods. Eating whole foods, those resembling the food's original form, is more nutritious because many nutrients (vitamins, minerals, fiber) may be lost in processing, and ingredients such as sugar, sodium, and fat may be added. As an example, using the same amount of calories for different forms of potatoes, a baked potato offers 20 milligrams of vitamin C, French fries contain 7 milligrams, while potato chips have 2 milligrams of vitamin C (Boyle and Zyla 1996). This doesn't mean you should never eat French fries or potato chips, but rather you should balance them with foods containing higher amounts of vitamin C and lower amounts of fat. Therefore, the ADA urges Americans to avoid the idea of "good foods" and "bad foods" (ADA 2002b). It is the position of the ADA that all foods can fit into a healthful eating style and healthy diet if consumed in moderation and combined with regular physical activity (ADA 2002b).

ACSM Recommendations on Nutrition

Five Ways to Eat Better
1. Eat a good breakfast every day.
    a. Eat fruits, low-fat milk, yogurt, and low-fat cheeses.
    b. Use a bran-type or fortified cereal for fiber and vitamins.
2. Get enough protein.
    a. Use skinless chicken, fish, and lean meats as main courses.
    b. Eat whole grains, nuts, seeds, peas, and beans daily.
    c. Eat low-fat dairy products daily; eggs occasionally.
3. Drink plenty of water.
    a. Fruit juices and Popsicles are good alternatives to water.
    b. Tea, coffee, and alcohol increase water loss. Try cocoa instead.
4. Fiber is important.
    a. Eat whole grain cereals and breads.
    b. Eat raw vegetables and fruits with skin.
    c. Add dry beans to soups and stews.
5. Minimize high sugar and processed foods.
    a. Sweets are high in calories and low in nutrients.
    b. Use table sugar and syrups in small amounts.

Five Reasons to Eat Well

1. Malnutrition presents a major health risk.
   a. One in four older Americans is undernourished.
   b. Malnutrition increases the likelihood of diseases.
2. Diet requirements change with aging.
   a. Taste and thirst decrease, so pay attention to water and food needs.
   b. Medication can affect appetite.
3. Medications may interact with foods.
   a. Ask your pharmacist/doctor how/if your medications will interact with food.
   b. Make careful food choices if on medication.
4. Vitamin and mineral deficiencies can be avoided.
   a. Careful food choices are essential.
   b. Select foods with high nutrient value.
5. Calorie needs increase with exercise.
   a. Exercise for successful aging.
   b. Daily exercise burns 100 to 400 calories and allows greater choices of healthy foods.

In the current USDA Food Guide, the latest recommendation is to eat 2 cups (4 servings) of fruit and 2.5 cups (5 servings) of vegetables per day, based on a 2,000 calorie diet (DGA 2005a). Selecting a variety of fruits and vegetables daily can bring potential health benefits related to cancer, obesity, heart diesease, and hypertension (ADA 2000). For more information about the Dietary Guidelines for Americans, go to www.healthierus.gov/ dietary guidelines.

To make healthy food choices you should know the serving size, nutrient content, and calories from fats, carbohydrates, and proteins. Food labels provide this information for all processed foods (refer to figure 7.1 on reading a food label), but fresh fruits and vegetables do not have a food label. Table 7.3 provides examples of serving sizes for the various food groups as well as recommended number of servings per day.

As you make your daily food choices, read the food labels. Learn what amount is considered a "serving" of the foods you eat. Many people misjudge the actual size of a serving. You could be consuming several servings in

Nutrition Facts

Serving Size 1 cup (59g)

Servings Per Container about 10

Amount Per Serving	Cereal	Cereal with 1/2 cup Fat-Free Milk
Calories	190	230
Calories from Fat	10	10
	% Daily Value**	
Total Fat 1 g*	2%	2%
Saturated Fat 0 g	0%	0%
Polyunsaturated Fat 0.5 g		
Monounsaturated Fat 0 g		
Cholesterol 0 mg	0%	0%
Sodium 360 mg	15%	18%
Potassium 360 mg	10%	16%
Total Carbohydrate 46 g	15%	17%
Dietary Fiber 8 g	32%	32%
Soluble Fiber 1 g		
Sugars 20 g		
Other Carbohydrate 18 g		
Protein 4 g		
Vitamin A	15%	20%
Vitamin C	0%	2%
Calcium	2%	15%
Iron	60%	60%
Vitamin D	10%	25%
Thiamin	25%	30%
Riboflavin	35%	35%
Niacin	35%	35%
Vitamin B-6	25%	25%
Folic Acid	25%	25%
Vitamin B-12	25%	35%
Phosphorus	20%	30%
Magnesium	20%	25%
Zinc	15%	20%
Copper	15%	15%

*Amount in Cereal; one-half cup fat-free milk contributes an additional 40 calories, 65 mg sodium, 200 mg potassium, 6 g total carbohydrate (6 g sugars), and 5 g protein.

**Percent Daily Values are based on a 2,000 calorie diet. Your daily values may be higher or lower depending on your calorie needs:

	Calories	2,000	2,500
Total Fat	Less than	65 g	85 g
Sat. Fat	Less than	20 g	25 g
Cholest	Less than	300 mg	300 mg
Sodium	Less than	2,400 mg	2,400 mg
Potassium		3,500 mg	3,500 mg
Total Carb		300 g	375 g
Fiber		35 g	30 g

Ingredients: Whole grain wheat, raisins, wheat bran, sugar, corn syrup, salt, wheat flour, malted barley flour, honey.
Vitamins and Minerals: Reduced iron, niacinamide, zinc oxide (source of zinc), vitamin B-6, vitamin A palmitate, riboflavin (vitamin B-2), thiamin mononitrate (vitamin B-1), folic acid, vitamin B-12, vitamin D.

Serving Size is set for foods. Doubling the servings doubles the percentages given for the Daily Value and doubles the calories.

Daily Value (DV) shows how this food fits into your daily diet. Daily values are set at 2,000 calories. Your caloric intake may be higher or lower than 2,000 calories. (5% DV or less is low; 20% DV or more is high.)

Total Fat lists all the fat grams and separates the three types of fat. Note that due to rounding, the total fat is not always a sum of the component parts.

Cholesterol and Sodium need to be limited in the daily diet.

Total Carbohydrate includes fiber, simple sugars, and other sugars (complex carbohydrates).

Protein does not show a % Daily Value because it requires expensive testing to determine.

Ingredients are listed in descending order of amounts.

Figure 7.1   Reading a food label.

Table 7.3   Examples of Serving Sizes

Food group	Recommended number of servings per day*	Examples of serving sizes
Fruit group	2 c = 4 servings (fresh, frozen, dried, canned—packed in own juice)	1 medium fruit 1/2 c berries or melon 1/4 c dried fruit 1/2 c 100% fruit juice
Vegetable group	2 1/2 c = 5 servings (fresh, frozen, or canned)	1/2 c cut-up raw or cooked vegetable 1 c raw leafy vegetable 1/2 cup vegetable juice
Grain group	6 oz equivalents	1 oz equivalent is • 1 slice bread • 1 c dry cereal • 1/2 c cooked rice, pasta, cereal
Meat and beans group	5.5 oz equivalents	1 oz equivalent is • 1 oz cooked lean meats, poultry, fish • 1 egg • 1/4 c cooked dry beans or tofu • 1 tbsp peanut butter • 1/2 oz nuts or seeds
Milk group	3 c	1 c equivalent is • 1 c low- or nonfat milk or yogurt • 1 1/2 oz low- or nonfat natural cheese • 2 oz low- or nonfat processed cheese
Oils	6 tsp	1 tsp equivalent is • 1 tbsp low-fat mayo • 2 tbsp light salad dressing • 1 tsp vegetable oil

*Based on a 2,000-calorie diet

Data reprinted from the Sample USDA Food Guide, Dietary Guidelines for Americans 2005, http://www.health.gov/dietaryguidelines/dga2005/document/pdf/Chapter2.pdf

a portion (the amount placed on a plate or bowl or in a glass or cup). For example, for breakfast you might have a glass of orange juice and a bowl of cereal with milk. How large was the glass of juice? Was it four ounces (1/2 cup), or did you fill a large glass and drink all the juice (several servings)? What size bowl did you use? Most people measure their portion by the size of bowl selected. Cereals vary in serving size from 1/3 cup to 1 1/2 cups. Did you eat a bagel for breakfast? How big was it? It could range from two to five servings of bread depending on its size. As you start to read food labels, you will become aware of the serving sizes and be less likely to unknowingly consume extra calories. It is easy to see why the ADA emphasizes portion control as a means of maintaining a healthy weight (ADA 2004).

Variety, Balance, and Moderation

These three words—*variety*, *balance*, and *moderation*—are the simple, direct recommendations of dietitians and health professionals. Most women get in the habit of eating their favorite foods, or eating what is available from vending machines and fast food chains, so they may be guilty of not eating a wide variety of foods. Different grains, fruits, vegetables, meats, and dairy foods can provide you with a wide assortment of nutrients. The colors, textures, and flavors of a wide variety of foods make food selections more interesting and healthy.

Balance refers to eating foods from all food groups rather than the majority from one or two food groups. Balance is also a matter of keeping your caloric intake adjusted to your caloric expenditure. Exercise for yourself. Enjoy the added benefit noted by very active women who often say part of the reason they exercise is so they can eat desserts or have their indulgences.

Moderation is the third key to healthy diet and life. Moderation refers to eating an appropriate serving size (ADA 2002b). Many Americans have difficulty understanding this concept. (Your mother or grandmother probably used to say, "All things in moderation.") The intake of fats, oils, and sweets is where almost everyone really needs to exercise self-control.

Dietary Guidelines for Americans

The current dietary guidelines for Americans include nine major messages (DGA 2005b):

1. Consume a variety of foods within and among the basic food groups while staying within energy needs.
2. Control caloric intake to manage body weight.
3. Be physically active every day.
4. Increase daily intake of fruits and vegetables, whole grains, and nonfat or low-fat milk and milk products.
5. Choose fats wisely for good health.
6. Choose carbohydrates wisely for good health.
7. Choose and prepare foods with little salt.
8. If you drink alcoholic beverages, do so in moderation.
9. Keep foods safe to eat.

Following these guidelines will help you maintain a healthy weight, encourage daily physical activities, and promote wholesome eating behaviors as well. It is entirely possible to remain healthy as you age, and your choices of activities and foods consumed can directly influence your physical ability to combat illness, handle stress, and prevent disease (Singh 2000).

Changing Nutritional Needs

As discussed previously, your nutritional needs change during perimenopause and postmenopause. Now more than ever, every calorie counts as you actively combat bone mineral loss and the possibility of creeping weight gain. Basically, your nutritional requirements are increasing at a time when your calorie requirements are decreasing (Singh 2000). This section explains how energy expenditure is determined and what your caloric intake should be.

Determining Energy Expenditure

Like a checking account, energy intake and energy expenditure require a balance. Unlike a bank, your body does not enforce stiff penalties for overdrafts; it simply loses weight or stores fat for future use. When you are neither losing nor gaining weight, your body is in a state of energy balance.

Three categories dictate your total daily energy expenditure: energy needed for the body at rest, energy required for physical activity, and energy necessary for the thermic effect of food (Williams 2002). Your basal metabolic rate (BMR) represents the amount of calories needed to sustain the functions of cells and tissues when the body is at rest (Williams 2002). BMR accounts for two-thirds of your daily energy expenditure (Singh 2000). Your physical activity level is the sum of all the movement, work, and exercise you perform in a day, whether in demanding, continuous, or slow activities. For a typical 60-year-old sedentary woman, the thermic effect of exercise (energy expenditure during and after physical activity) is 23 percent of her calories (Singh 2000). Last, the thermic effect of food (the process of digesting, absorbing, utilizing, and storing the food that has been eaten) requires between 5 and 10 percent of your daily calories (Williams 2002).

As you age, metabolism slows, muscle mass and metabolically active tissue are lost, and physical activity levels gradually decrease. This is why physical activity is such a critical part of the energy equation. No matter what your age, exercise causes the metabolic rate to increase. The more physically active you are, and the more lean muscle tissue you possess, the better you are able to control your weight. (Reread chapter 4 if necessary.) There just is no downside to a sensible, active lifestyle!

Caloric Requirements for Middle-Aged and Older Women

A number of factors influence your daily energy requirements. Beyond your physical activity level, age, and percentage of body fat, the other factors include gender, body weight, genetics, and disease (Singh 2000).

In general, "1200 to 1600 calories are about right for most inactive to moderately active older women, 1800 to 2200 calories are about right for active to very active older women, [and] 2400 to 2800 calories are about right for extremely active older women" (Singh 2000, 134). Table 7.4 is more specific regarding the number of daily calories needed for women at age 55. Using this table, you can find your body weight and physical activity level and better determine your daily energy needs.

Table 7.4 Expected Total Energy Requirements for Women at Age 55

Weight (lb)	Basal metabolism	Light activity*	Moderate activity**	Heavy activity***
100	1224	1714	1958	2203
110	1264	1770	2022	2275
120	1304	1826	2086	2347
130	1343	1880	2149	2417
140	1383	1936	2213	2489
150	1422	1991	2275	2560
160	1462	2047	2339	2632
170	1501	2104	2402	2702
180	1541	2157	2466	2774
190	1580	2212	2528	2844
200	1620	2268	2592	2916
210	1659	2323	2654	2986
220	1699	2379	2718	3058
230	1739	2435	2782	3130
240	1778	2489	2845	3200
250	1818	2525	2909	3272

*Light activity: does not perform regular vigorous exercise, walk for exercise, or climb stairs

**Moderate activity: performs moderate exercise (walking, dancing, gardening, swimming, biking) several times per week

***Heavy activity: participates in regular vigorous exercise (jogging, singles tennis, high-intensity weightlifting, stair stepping, powerwalking) several times per week

Calcium and Vitamin D

Calcium is a mineral needed in the body for many purposes, including bone health. Most of the calcium in the body is found in the bones, and it is calcium that gives strength to bones. Given the importance of calcium, you might expect that most women would be sure to consume adequate amounts. Unfortunately, up to 75 percent of women do not consume the recommended amounts of calcium (Williams 2002). To compound the problem of inadequate intake, estrogen is needed to maintain calcium balance in the body. As mentioned previously, estrogen levels decline at menopause, and thus calcium may be lost from the bones. Since calcium provides strength to the bones, the menopausal woman is more prone to fractures—in particular in the spine, at the end of the radius bone in the forearm by the wrist, and in the neck of the femur (thigh bone) at the hip (Williams 2002). Trabecular bone is found at these locations; categorized as "spongy bone" because of its more open lattice-type structure, it is the type of bone most affected by calcium deficiency. Trabecular bone actually starts its downward trend during one's 30s; decreases in cortical bone (the outer layer of bone) do not appear to begin until menopause (ACSM 1995).

The need for calcium and vitamin D go hand in hand. Calcium is an important component of bone, but in order to fulfill that role, it must be absorbed from the intestine and moved into the blood for delivery to the bones. Vitamin D helps the body absorb calcium from the intestines and is involved with calcium balance in the body. Calcium balance involves calcium intake and absorption as well as calcium excretion. The goal of positive calcium balance can be hampered by diets high in protein, caffeine, phosphorus, or sodium (Wilson 2003).

Calcium consumption in the diet can include dairy products, cheese, yogurt, dark green leafy vegetables, legumes, nuts, and calcium-fortified products (Williams 2002). In addition, people may use supplements to reach the target goal of 1,200 to 1,500 milligrams of calcium per day. When selecting a supplement, consider the form of the calcium (all contain calcium "salts"—meaning the calcium is linked with another substance). One of the better absorbed calcium supplements is calcium citrate (Williams 2002). It is also recommended that you consume the supplement in multiple small doses (i.e., three doses of 200 milligrams each with meals rather than one 600-milligram tablet); absorption is higher when the amount consumed is spread throughout the day rather than taken in one large dose (McClung 2003). In addition, avoid taking your calcium supplement with fiber or iron supplements. We would not recommend supplementing beyond a total of 600 milligrams per day because excessive amounts may contribute to heart contraction abnormalities, constipation, and, in some with family history, kidney stone development (Williams 2002). The daily recommendation for calcium is provided in table 7.5.

Vitamin D is not widely found in foods, although it is found in fortified foods such as milk. Exposure of the skin to sunlight also allows the body to form vitamin D. Ultraviolet-B radiation promotes vitamin D formation but, unfortunately, also causes wrinkles and skin cancer, so lengthy exposure to the sun is not recommended. It appears that 10 to 20 minutes of summer sunshine two or three times per week provides the recommended amounts of vitamin D (Williams 2002). During the winter, and in the northern parts of the world, it may be hard to get the recommended amount of vitamin D from sunshine (adequate intake is 400 IU for ages 51-70 and 600 IU for those over 70 years of age), so ensuring the diet also contains vitamin D is a good idea.

Both deficiencies and excesses of vitamin D can cause health problems. Excessive amounts of vitamin D increase calcium absorption and are deposited in the kidneys, potentially leading to kidney stones (Boyle and Zyla 1996). Vitamin D is a fat-soluble vitamin and is stored in the body, so take supplementation of this vitamin only on a physician's orders. (Refer to table 7.5 for the recommended daily intake of Vitamin D.)

Table 7.5 Recommended Daily Intake of Calcium and Vitamin D for Women

Daily recommendation for calcium*	
Age	**mg/day**
25-50	1,000
Pregnant or nursing	1,200-1,500
Over 50 (postmenopausal)	1,500
On estrogens	1,000
Not on estrogens	1,500
Over 65	1,500
Daily recommendation for vitamin D*	
Age	**International units (IUs)**
51-70	400
Over 70	600

*Calcium data from National Institutes of Health, 1994. "Optimal Calcium Intake." NIH Consensus Statement Online. National Institutes of Health, 12(4):1-31.

**Vitamin D data from ACOG 2003d.

Since this book deals primarily with the benefits of exercise on menopause, this section on nutrition provides only a simple overview. For more information on calcium, take the Women's Healthy Bone Quiz on the Internet at www.eatright.org. For further guidance on all aspects of nutrition, we recommend reading *Nancy Clark's Sports Nutrition Guidebook, Third Edition* (2003, Human Kinetics).

Managing Stress

The rest of this chapter moves away from nutrition and examines other ways to balance health and lifestyle practices during the journey through the menopause years. In this section, stress will be discussed and suggestions provided for ways to handle the physiological changes occurring in the body. Managing stress is beneficial to our overall health since we live with stress every day—situations at work and with family and friends. Handling your responses to stress in positive ways allows you the opportunity to thrive rather than to simply cope with stress.

Understanding Stress and Your Responses

Stress is known as a nonspecific response of the body to demands made on it. If you think about it, you do respond in imprecise ways to stress: your stomach flip-flops, your breathing increases, your palms moisten, and your heart beats rapidly.

Negative stressors and stress (your responses) are what cause so much difficulty. What stresses you may not even bother your friends, family, or coworkers. Stress can be divided into acute, episodic, and chronic situations (Hales and Zartman 2001). Acute stressors pop up any time, such as a flat tire, a broken bone, or narrowly avoiding an accident. They are quick, yet they cause a powerful physical response. Episodic stress is like a revolving door; it keeps coming around. It could include the monthly budget or annual reports, a difficult coworker, or handling hot flashes while on the job. These incidences occur periodically and temporarily raise stress levels. Chronic stressors may be the most damaging because they are long term, affecting you physically, mentally, and emotionally. Examples include living with a chronic illness or overloads at work or home.

The stress response of the body is as ancient as primitive men and women. When in danger, they needed the "fight or flight" response—to fight a predator or flee and live another day. To this day your body's stress response is the same as that of a caveman: Your heart races, muscles tense, breathing increases, your brain is alert, digestion stops, and many chemicals and hormones are dumped into the bloodstream to help you defeat your foe. The problem in modern society is that there is no bear or lion to fight or flee, but your stress response is the same. Unfortunately, the stress hormones stay in the blood for hours. Under chronic stress, the elevated levels of stress hormones raise insulin levels, increase the body fat of inactive people, and are a partial contributor of atherosclerotic plaque in the coronary arteries (Hales and Zartman 2001).

As you deal with multiple sources of stress in your life—both negative and positive—you still need to be able to function well. The trick is to have just enough stress in your life to keep you motivated, but not so much that you are overloaded.

Practicing Stress Management Techniques

The great thing about aging is the experience and wisdom of living life. Put events and situations in perspective with what is most important to you. Let's take a look at some of the most productive methods to manage stress.

Of course, first on our list is exercise. It is the closest way to channel the original "fight or flight" response. Lots of otherwise unused aggression or anger can be controlled when jogging, swimming, walking, or whacking a tennis or golf ball. After exercise your mind will be clearer, and with regular exercise your next response to stress will be milder (Fahey, Insel, and Roth 2003).

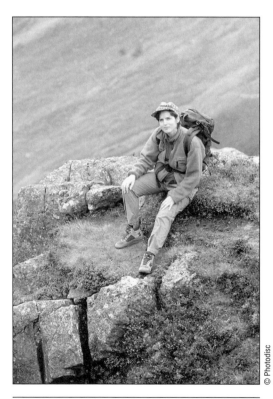

Another top-of-our list stress management technique is re-evaluation. Stop and clearly evaluate and consider your priorities, obligations, and schedule. Prioritize. What is most important to you? What can take a back seat? In what commitments must you really be involved? Can you excuse yourself from the minor ones? Look for ways to downsize your schedule, then guard it from future overload. (Caution: This takes practice!)

Use positive mental imagery and positive self-talk. Rather than see yourself doing something poorly, imagine succeeding and completing this task with flair and grace. Listen to your personal self-talk. If you

Take an invigorating hike. Enjoy the outdoors and leave your worries behind.

hear yourself saying, "You're so stupid," or "Dummy," then stop it. Replace these harmful thoughts with praise for your efforts and behaviors. Changing your mental images and self-talk to positive affirmations can change the way you view situations.

Talk to trusted individuals. When was the last time you had a heart-to-heart talk with your significant other or best friend? Lay it out and then listen. Usually this discussion can give you a different perspective, or at least you will feel better by expressing yourself. Knowing that someone cares enough to listen always helps. Often, your spouse or good friends can help you see the lighter side and get you to laugh at the situation or yourself.

Cultivate your interests and hobbies. Haven't had the time during the last 10 to 20 years? Start doing the activities you enjoy. Read. Garden. Bake. Dance. Draw. Fish. Play with your pet. Play a musical instrument. Join an activity-type club or group so you can socialize and enjoy your hobby (pinochle group, ski club), or take an adult education class if you've always wanted to learn to sew, paint, play the piano, or do woodworking. Adults often forget how to play, so let your interests and hobbies help you remember.

Other commonsense stress busters include the following:

- Listen to music. It doesn't matter what kind. Belt out the lyrics or hum along. Lose yourself in the melody or the chorus. Music stimulates your brain yet can comfort you and reduce your blood pressure and muscle tension.

- Take five. When you are angry or sad, go someplace where you can be alone. Take five minutes and let your emotions out. Feel sorry for yourself, and be done with it. Then, continue your earlier activities.

- Breathe. Practice controlled breathing—deep, slow inhalations. Place one hand on your abdomen and the other hand on your chest. Inhale through your nose, and allow your abdomen to move instead of your chest. Exhale slowly through your mouth. Focus on your breathing for 5 to 10 minutes.

- Keep a journal or diary to express your feelings and review your problems.

- Get a massage. Whether a full-body or a shoulder or foot massage, the result is reduced muscle tension and anxiety.

- Try meditation, yoga, or tai chi for controlled breathing, stretching, and exercise.

- Take care of yourself. Get enough sleep each night. Eat healthy, nutrient-dense foods. Limit your intake of caffeine, salt, sugar, and alcohol. And, finally, laugh out loud several times every day.

Maintaining Sexual Health

There is no set age when sexual feelings cease (Singh 2000). You have been a sexual being throughout your life, and changing hormone levels do not mean you cannot continue to be sexual. Beyond hormonal changes that begin before and continue through menopause, a woman's sexuality is related to physical and emotional health, stress, strengths and weaknesses of the intimate relationship (Singh 2000), sexual desire, ability to respond sexually, and feelings of attractiveness (Beach 1976). Two-thirds of men and women surveyed by the American Association of Retired Persons (AARP) reported that they are satisfied with their sex lives (Jacoby 1999). At midlife, many women feel liberated by menopause because they no longer need to worry about pregnancy or contraception.

Physiological Changes Before and After Menopause

From the perimenopause years to the postmenopause years, your body will undergo many physiological changes. These changes may present both challenges and opportunities in your lovemaking (Midlife sexuality and women 2004). As estrogen production from your ovaries declines during perimenopause and then stops during menopause, you may experience the following changes in your sexual health (Midlife sexuality and women 2004):

- Vaginal changes including decreased lubrication and a narrowing of the vaginal opening, which can lead to painful intercourse, or dyspareunia (pronounced DIS-puh-ROO-ne-uh).

- Diminished or slowed sexual response due to decreased blood flow to the genitals.

- Changes in sensitivity due to thinning of the vaginal walls and greater exposure of the clitoris.

- Higher risk of infections due to changes in vaginal walls and a change in vaginal acidity, causing an increased potential for tissue damage and bacterial or yeast infections.

- Stress incontinence due to changes in the urethral sphincter caused by reduced estrogen. This may cause urine leaks during intercourse.

With continued sexual activity, postmenopausal women report having less painful intercourse and fewer problems with vaginal lubrication (Singh 2000). Because arousal and lubrication take longer after menopause, plan on longer foreplay in order to avoid painful lovemaking.

Sexual desire, or libido, can diminish during menopause for a variety of reasons. Reduced lubrication and reduced elasticity of the vaginal walls contributing to dyspareunia may be a primary reason for avoiding sex. The side effects of menopause (hot flashes, night sweats, sleeplessness, and irritability) may also become distracters to sexual enjoyment (Midlife sexuality and women 2004). During this time in your life, it is important to maintain your annual gynecological exams so your physician can treat you for the most bothersome perimenopausal symptoms.

Communicate honestly with your partner, who may be experiencing similar feelings of inhibition or reluctance for lovemaking because of age and hormonal changes. Offset vaginal dryness by using over-the-counter lubricants and vaginal moisturizers. There are a variety of water-based brands: K-Y Jelly, Astroglide, GyneMoistrin, Lubrin inserts, Moist Again, and Vagisil Intimate Moisturizer (ACOG 2003a). Always use water-based lubricants because petroleum-based products increase the possibility of vaginal infections and may damage latex condoms and diaphragms (ACOG 2003a). For nonsmoking perimenopausal women needing contraception, consider low-dose oral contraceptives to reduce vaginal dryness (ACOG 2003a). K-Y Plus and Advantage 24 are water-based lubricants that also contain spermicide (ACOG 2003a).

Perimenopause Contraception

Perimenopause and menopause are fairly simple to define but are tricky in terms of actual contraception. By definition, perimenopause can last about four years and continues 12 months after your last period (NIH 2001a). Your menstrual cycles will become irregular, so natural family planning methods will make it very difficult for you to accurately predict ovulation. Continue to use a reliable form of contraception until your physician concludes that you are past menopause. Remember, the use of oral contraceptives may relieve some perimenopausal symptoms such as vaginal dryness and hot flashes but will cause the regular continuation of your periods even after you have passed menopause (NIH 2001a).

Prevention of Sexually Transmitted Diseases

Although the menopause years may make sex more carefree because of freedom from pregnancy, sexually transmitted diseases (STDs) are still possible. Sadly, many menopausal women have contracted HIV/AIDS and other STDs because they felt sexually liberated and did not use barrier protection during sex. Postmenopausal women face an even greater risk for HIV infection because of the fragility and thinning of the vaginal walls (NIH 2001a). When having sex with a new partner, or if you are not in a mutual long-term monogamous relationship, always use a barrier of a latex condom lubricated with spermicide to reduce the transmission rate of STDs.

Continuing Health Examinations and Tests

As with other stages in your life, it is very important that you continue to take care of yourself. You still need regular gynecological examinations, recommended age-related medical tests, and immunizations. For some health conditions, such as cervical cancer, the rate of incidence increases as you age (ACOG 2003b). Additionally, after age 50, there is more urgency for mammograms, screening tests for colon cancer, and blood tests for thyroid-stimulating hormone. As you become menopausal, the changing hormonal levels put you at increased risk for cardiovascular diseases. This section provides a general list of the medical examinations and tests you need during the menopausal years.

Pap Tests and Pelvic Exams

Pap tests have long been the best diagnostic screening for cervical cancer. Certain strains of the *human papillomavirus* (HPV) and genital warts are primary risk factors for cervical cancer. A new version of the Pap test—the HPV-DNA test, which examines DNA (genetic material)—can identify the presence of high-risk HPV as well as any other cervical cell changes (ACOG 2003b). ACOG has released the following new screening guidelines for women over age 30 (ACOG 2003b, 8):

- Pap tests. With normal results of three consecutive annual Pap tests, your physician's advice may be a two- or three-year interval for subsequent Pap tests.
- Pap tests combined with HPA-DNA tests. When both the Pap test and the HPA-DNA test are negative, you will be rescreened with the combined tests every three years. More frequent screening will occur when one of these tests is positive. If you are HIV positive, are immunosuppressed from an organ transplant, are a DES daughter (exposed to DES, a carcinogen, in utero), or have previously been diagnosed with cervical cancer, more frequent screenings will be needed.

If you have had a hysterectomy or the removal of your cervix along with your uterus for noncancerous reasons, your physician may recommend no further Pap tests. With a hysterectomy and a previous history of abnormal cell growth, you will be screened annually until there are three negative tests. As with other medical decisions, a variety of personal issues must be taken into consideration regarding the continuation or cessation of cervical screening tests.

After age 45, the ACOG recommends that all women receive an annual pelvic examination to determine the health of their reproductive organs (ACOG 2003c). Most commonly, the pelvic exam is performed during the same gynecological visit as the Pap test. Before your annual exam, prepare a list of questions to ask your gynecologist about any concerns or annoying symptoms you have experienced. This is a great time to ask questions about your sexual health and get advice or explanations.

Mammograms

Mammograms still remain the best screening tool for detecting breast cancer. The ACOG recommends women in their 40s receive mammograms every one or two years, while women in their 50s have annual mammograms. For more information regarding mammograms and for mammography facilities in your area, call 1-800-4-CANCER. Additionally, the National Cancer Institute maintains an extensive website on breast cancer screening and information at cancernet.nci.nih.gov/pat_home.htm (NIH 1997).

In addition to mammograms, women should always perform a breast self-examination on a monthly basis as a line of defense between mammograms. Although a mammogram will detect small lumps much sooner than you can by self-exam, in between your annual mammograms, you can find small lumps that may appear. For your breast self-exams, select a date of the month you can remember, then perform them on this day every month.

Bone Density Checks

Tests to measure your bone strength are called bone densitometry or bone mineral density (BMD) tests (Bone density testing 2004). Bone density checks are recommended for all women over the age of 65, for menopausal women with recent bone fractures, and for younger women with osteoporosis risk factors (Bone density testing 2004). Unlike many other medical tests, the BMD tests are noninvasive and pain-free.

Various tests are available for BMD measurement, with different levels of accuracy and expense. Generally, drugstores and temporary locations use the smaller and portable units known as peripheral devices. Peripheral devices measure the bone density in a finger or heel, and these tests cost much less than BMD tests measuring the bones of the hip and spine (Bone density testing 2004). Peripheral bone tests are not as accurate for predicting the major debilitating fractures that osteoporosis causes—those of the spine or hip. Central devices measure the bone density in the spine or hip and are the most accurate. They include the following tests (Bone density testing 2004):

- Dual energy X-ray absorptiometry (DEXA), the most accurate test available, is able to detect a 1 percent bone density change in your spine or hip. For this test, you lie on a platform while a mechanical imager moves over your body. The DEXA test produces about one-tenth the radiation of a chest X ray.

- Quantitative computerized tomography (QCT) emits more radiation than the DEXA scans while providing a three-dimensional image of your bones. The QCT test measures the BMD of the spine while you lie on a table that is moved into a tubelike area, where the image is produced. It takes about 10 minutes to perform this test.

Bone density tests are typically reported in T-scores. The T-score is a comparison of your bone density with that of a young, healthy female (Bone density testing 2004). T-scores are units—standard deviations—above or below a set standard (Bone density testing 2004). The World Health Organization suggests the following levels for interpretation of T-scores (Bone density testing 2004):

- Above –1: This is a normal bone density.
- Between –1 and –2.5: This score is a sign of osteopenia (a pre-osteoporosis condition). Your bone density is below normal.
- Below –2.5: You have osteoporosis.

A low BMD score is a strong predictor of the risk of an osteoporosis-related fracture (National Osteoporosis Foundation 2002). Maintaining your bone health requires the following measures: receiving enough dietary calcium, maintaining your muscular strength through weight-bearing activities, not smoking or using alcohol excessively, and getting routine BMD tests (National Osteoporosis Foundation 2002).

Cholesterol (Lipid) Tests

After age 20, you should have a fasting blood lipid test (total cholesterol, LDL, HDL, and triglyceride) once every five years (AHA 2004a). This blood test will require you to fast for 12 to 14 hours (nonfasting tests are less accurate). After menopause, the low-density lipoprotein (LDL) level in women is likely to increase because of the reduction in available estrogen (Singh 2000). Reducing your LDL cholesterol can lower the chance of heart attacks and strokes (National Cholesterol Education Program 1993). If the LDL level remains elevated, physicians will usually recommend making dietary adjustments in order to reduce it (Singh 2000). These dietary changes would include reducing calories from fat intake, specifically targeting saturated fats. The classifications for total and LDL blood cholesterol levels are listed in table 7.6 (NIH 2001b).

High-density lipoprotein (HDL) cholesterol is the "good" cholesterol that reduces the risk of cardiovascular disease. It ranges from 50 to 60 mg/dL in the average woman (AHA 2004). An HDL cholesterol level less than 40 mg/dL is low, increasing the risk of heart disease. After menopause, the HDL level will decrease because of the reduction of female sex hormones (AHA 2004). Being physically active, maintaining a healthy weight, and not smoking are three ways to raise a low HDL level (AHA 2004).

Table 7.6 Classifications of Blood Cholesterol Levels

Total cholesterol (mg/dL)	LDL cholesterol (mg/dL)
Desirable: Lower than 200	Optimal: Lower than 100
Borderline high: 200-239	Near optimal/above optimal: 100-129
High risk: 240 or higher	Borderline high: 130-159
	High: 160-189
	Very high: 190 or higher

Data from "The Third Report of the National Cholesterol Education Program Expert Panel on Detection, Evaluation, and Treatment of High Blood Cholesterol in Adults." NIH Publication, No. 01-3670, May 2001, p. 3.

A quality blood cholesterol test also provides a cholesterol ratio. The ratio is calculated by dividing the total cholesterol level by the HDL cholesterol level. The lower the ratio, the better it is. Keep the ratio below 5: 1; with the optimal ratio at 3.5:1 (AHA 2004).

Blood Pressure Tests

Your blood pressure is a measure of the pressure your heart exerts on your arteries when contracting (systolic pressure) and between beats (diastolic pressure). Your blood pressure should be checked at least once a year. Table 7.7 provides the blood pressure classifications (NIH 2003). Although blood pressure varies during the day with activity level, healthy adults should have a blood pressure reading of less than 120/80 (NIH 2003).

Table 7.7 Classification of Blood Pressure for Adults (Age 18 and Older)

Blood pressure category	Systolic blood pressure (mm Hg)	Diastolic blood pressure (mm Hg)
Normal	Lower than 120	and lower than 80
Prehypertension	120-139	or 80-89
Stage 1 hypertension	140-159	or 90-99
Stage 2 hypertension	160 or higher	or 100 or higher

Accurate classification of blood pressure is based on 2 or more properly measured, seated blood pressure readings from 2 or more visits to the office of a health professional.

Data from "The Seventh Report of the Joint National Committee on Prevention, Detection, Evaluation, and Treatment of High Blood Pressure." NIH Publication, No. 03-5233, May 2003, p. 2-3.

Menopause seems to cause a 5 mmHg increase in the systolic pressure of women that is unrelated to the effects of aging and gaining weight (Staessen et al. 1997). After age 45, the ACOG (2003c) recommends that women receive annual blood pressure testing if their blood pressure is 140/90 or higher.

Physical activity is good for every woman's blood pressure, whether in the normal or hypertensive range. According to the ACSM (1999), regular exercise (30 minutes or more) usually decreases both the systolic and diastolic values of the blood pressure within three to four weeks. Physical fitness level is a major determinant of keeping your blood pressure under control in middle and older age (ACSM 1999). This demonstrates another strong reason why exercise is or should be important in your life as you deal with menopause.

If you purchase an automatic blood pressure kit to monitor your own blood pressure at home, take it with you to your next doctor's appointment. Ask your physician to check your blood pressure machine against the professional blood pressure unit to verify the accuracy of the reading. Many people get "white coat hypertension," which means their blood pressure rises when they are in the doctor's office. Keeping a home journal of your blood pressure readings can be very useful to your physician, so take your blood pressure journal with you to your medical appointments.

Thyroid Check

After age 35, have your thyroid checked every five years with a thyroid-stimulating hormone (TSH) blood test (American Thyroid Association [ATA] 2004). The thyroid is a butterfly-shaped gland near the lower half of your throat and above your collarbone. Your thyroid creates hormones that regulate the physical and chemical processes of almost all organs and cells in your body. An underactive thyroid can produce symptoms of fatigue, mood swings, mild weight gain, forgetfulness, depression, and dry skin and hair (ATA 2004). Conversely, the opposite symptoms occur with an overactive thyroid: weight loss, diarrhea, difficulty sleeping, and excessive sweating. Low levels of TSH are associated with raising your total cholesterol and a slight increase in your blood pressure, while high TSH levels can decrease bone mineral density (ATA 2004). TSH blood tests can identify early stages of thyroid disease so treatment can be initiated (ATA 2004).

Other Screening Tests and Immunizations

Other tests and immunizations you may want to discuss with your physician include but are not limited to the following:

- Blood glucose tests: every 3 to 5 years
- Eye examinations: annually, with a check for glaucoma

- Colon cancer check: without family risk of colon cancer, an initial colonoscopy after age 50, repeated every 10 years, or a flexible sigmoidoscopy every 5 years (American Cancer Society 2004)
- Skin cancer check: annually
- Immunizations: annual influenza shot; pneumonia vaccination once every 5 years after age 50; a booster tetanus shot every 7 to 10 years

Summary

After reading this chapter you should have a better understanding of the need to take care of yourself for continued good health. Following the suggestions in this chapter will help you balance your body's changing needs as you successfully move from perimenopause into the postmenopausal years. Instead of viewing menopause as a negative time, utilize your crone wisdom and live this stage of your life as the French might recommend: with a "joie de vivre" (joy of living).

ACTION PLAN:

BALANCING EXERCISE, NUTRITION, AND STRESS

☐ Compare your food intake with recommended amounts for your age, sex, and activity level:
- Determine the number of servings you eat for each food group.
- Plan for improvements where you note excess or deficient numbers of servings.

☐ Read food labels, and make nutrient-dense choices.

☐ Evaluate your stressors, and work to decrease the stress in your life.

☐ Protect your health:
- Continue your regular mammograms and gynecological exams.
- Consider a bone density test.
- Monitor blood pressure and cholesterol levels.
- Schedule screening tests for thyroid-stimulating hormone, blood glucose, colon cancer, and skin cancer.

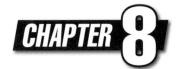

MAINTAINING YOUR
MOTIVATION

Y ou have arrived at chapter 8—congratulations! The previous chapters
equipped you with information to create an effective and realistic
workout program as you move through menopause. Maintaining
your momentum will require some planning. Simply knowing what to do
is not the same as implementing that knowledge on a daily and weekly
basis. The American College of Sports Medicine (2000) notes dropout
rates from exercise programs range from 9 to 87 percent. The first three
months of an exercise program are critical because dropout is highest
during that period. We present these findings not to discourage you but
rather to give you an honest look at the challenge. We will not try to hide
the truth—your exercise program *will* take time and effort. You need to
deliberately decide to make it a priority. If you read the preceding chapters,
you are aware of the health benefits, and you know how to begin or how
to improve what you have already started. Chapter 2 included a discussion of establishing goals. You now possess the knowledge and tools to
write your specific short-term and long-term goals. Figure 8.1 includes
a goal-setting worksheet to allow you to specifically address long-term
and short-term exercise goals as well as how you will handle obstacles to
reaching your goals. This chapter focuses on ways to complement those
goals and ensure you maintain your motivation.

In the spaces below, write your goals for your exercise plan in measurable terms. List dates or times to make the goals more specific.

Long-Term Goal(s)

An example of a long-term goal for cardiorespiratory fitness would be: Complete a 5K walk/run on (date).

   1. Cardiorespiratory fitness: _____

         _____

         _____

   2. Muscular strength and endurance: _____

         _____

         _____

   3. Flexibility: _____

         _____

Short-Term Goals

Specific short-term goals divide your long-term goal(s) into workable segments and should be updated monthly. Check the box below (and date it) when the short-term goal has been reached.

Month: _____

   1. Cardiorespiratory fitness: _____

         _____

   2. Muscular fitness: _____ ☐ _____

         _____

   3. Flexibility: _____ ☐ _____

         _____

Possible Obstacles to Reaching My Goal(s) Include ☐

_____

_____

_____

Ways to Overcome These Obstacles Include

_____

_____

_____

People Who Will Help Me Reach My Long-Term Goals Include

   1. _____   3. _____

   2. _____   4. _____

_____   _____
       (your signature)   (date)

Figure 8.1 Worksheet for exercise goals.

From *Action Plan for Menopause* by Barbara Bushman and Janice Clark Young, 2005, Champaign, IL: Human Kinetics.

Planning Ahead

You have established a plan that includes cardiorespiratory conditioning, muscular conditioning, and flexibility exercises. Charting your plan for the future, including involvement of family and friends, will help keep you on course.

Activity Logs

An activity log is like an exercise diary. We have included an example in table 8.1 of a very simple log to chart progress in all three key areas. Within the other chapters, exercise-specific charts are included for your use. Your activity log can be as general or specific as you want it to be. It is helpful to keep a daily record of all your exercise activities (cardiorespiratory, muscular, or stretching), comments about how you felt that day, and any other pertinent information (e.g., heart rate, health status, environmental conditions, or other conflicting priorities).

Some women write their exercise activities in their schedule books, while others maintain a separate notebook. If you have a computer, you may want to sign up for free activity charting. Various groups offer resources at no cost on their Web sites. One example is the American Heart Association. They offer a wonderful program called Just Move, which can be found at www.justmove.org/home.cfm. At this site, click on the Exercise Diary and create a password. Then, you will be prompted to enter your exercise goals for a 6-, 8-, or 12-week period to create your customized log.

Keeping a log allows you to reflect on your progress as well as the balance in your program. You may find that you have neglected stretching for a week or that you have reached a plateau in your strength training. In this way, the log can serve as a reminder to keep balance in your program. Remind yourself of the following ACSM guidelines:

- Cardiorespiratory conditioning → three to five days per week
- Muscular strength and endurance → two to three days per week
- Flexibility exercises → two to three days per week

These are overall guidelines to follow, allowing you to individualize your program within the recommended ranges.

Family Plan

The involvement of family and friends in your exercise program may seem superfluous, but research suggests it is vital to be successful. Spouse and peer approval are associated with good adherence to an exercise program (ACSM 2000). Without support of those closest to you, it might be difficult to maintain your focus. A physically active lifestyle benefits *everyone*.

Table 8.1   Sample Activity Log for Comprehensive Program

Day	C—M—F*	Time or distance	Comments (heart rate, rating of perceived exertion, health status, environmental conditions, and so on)
Sunday			
Monday			
Tuesday			
Wednesday			
Thursday			
Friday			
Saturday			
Weekly summary	C ➔ # workouts =	# minutes =	
	M ➔ # workouts =	# minutes =	
	F ➔ # workouts =	# minutes =	
Next week's goal:			

*C = cardiorespiratory; **M** = muscular; **F** = flexibility

From *Action Plan for Menopause* by Barbara Bushman and Janice Clark Young, 2005, Champaign, IL: Human Kinetics.

Please recall some of the take-home points from the Surgeon General's Report on Physical Activity and Health (US DHHS 1996):

- Approximately two-thirds of American adults are not achieving the recommended amount of physical activity (and one-fourth are totally inactive).
- People become more inactive as they age.
- Inactivity is higher in women than in men.
- Almost 50 percent of young people between 12 and 21 years of age are not vigorously active on a regular basis.

- Physical activity levels drop sharply during adolescence (and girls are less active than boys).

Thus, activity is important not only for you but also for your family and others who surround you. We encourage you to include family and peers in building a mutually supportive network so all can benefit from regular physical activity.

Adherence Pledge

As discussed in chapter 2, setbacks in any program will happen. Although setbacks are not part of your plan, your response to setbacks can and should be preplanned. Following is a sample pledge for you to use or modify to help you stick with your exercise program.

I pledge to put my health as a number one priority in my weekly schedule.

I will chart my workouts daily and reflect on my progress at the end of each month.

I pledge to update my short-term goals on the first day of each month.

You can add additional lines to the pledge specific to your health and wellness goals. You might want to print the pledge and place it somewhere you will regularly see it and be reminded of its importance in your life. Mark your calendar with monthly reminders to check your progress and to establish updated short-term goals.

Finding Programs That Work for You

In establishing your personal exercise goals, location and resources are central considerations. We discuss several options here, realizing each woman has her own preferences and unique opportunities. You may find a combination of programs works best for you.

Organized Programs

Most communities offer a variety of organized exercise programs. These can include community recreation programs, mall walkers, hiking clubs, biking clubs, master's groups (swimming, jogging), and exercise groups at your apartment, subdivision, or workplace. These programs may vary in level of organization and offerings. Evaluate your needs, your interests, and what is convenient for you. Some programs may be free and one-dimensional (e.g., mall walkers), while others offer a variety of exercise modes and opportunities (community recreation and worksite programs) for a given time period (4 to 12 weeks). Others may require an annual membership (e.g., biking clubs). Learn what is available in your community, and consider the many exercise possibilities.

Health Clubs

Joining a health club provides you with many options for your workouts. Treadmills, stationary bikes, stair steppers, a pool, and other equipment are typically available for cardiorespiratory endurance training. In addition, free weights as well as machines are usually available for muscular strength and endurance training. The amount and variety of equipment and scheduled classes available make joining a health club an attractive option.

When selecting a health club, you should consider several factors:

- Location. Is the facility located in a safe and easily accessible area? Is it near your workplace or home?

- Hours of operation. Is the facility open during the times of day you are available to exercise? If you enjoy an early morning swim, is the pool open during that time? Is the club closed on the weekends or over holidays? Will your membership give you unlimited access to the facility (i.e., no limit to the number of times you can work out in a week)?

- Equipment availability. Take a complete tour of the facility. Is the equipment clean and in good repair? Are your preferred pieces of equipment available? Visit the facility at a time when you would typically exercise. Is it overly crowded at that time? Is there enough equipment available, or are people waiting in line for access?

- Supervision. Ask about the credentials of the staff. At a minimum, staff should be certified in CPR and first aid. For personal trainers, an advanced certification is a must (see the sidebar on page 191 for more information). Is there a posted and practiced emergency plan? Is an automated external defibrillator (AED) available in case of a cardiac arrest? Is the staff available for questions regarding use of various pieces of equipment?

- Locker rooms. Are the locker rooms clean? Are the shower facilities well maintained and clean? Is a towel service available?

- Pool. Is there always a lifeguard on deck during open hours? Does the lifeguard maintain a continued focus on the patrons in the water? Is the water quality good (e.g., water should be clear and at an appropriate temperature)?

- Member services. Does the club offer special programs that may serve as an incentive to remain active (e.g., charting miles walked to earn points for some reward)? Are there special classes that interest you (e.g., water aerobics or spinning classes)? Are instructors for those courses qualified and trained? If needed, is child care provided? Is there a women-only section of the facility? (Note: Some women enjoy this option, while for others it is not an issue.)

When selecting a health club, treat it as you would the interview process for a job. Make sure it is the best environment and the best fit for you. Do not feel pressured to join during your first meeting or tour of the facility. There are many options, so you should shop around.

Personal Trainers

You may decide to use a personal trainer to assist you with your exercise program. A trainer can typically be employed through the health club or on a private basis in your home. Some women find a trainer helps solidify their commitment and motivation for their exercise programs. For more information on selecting a qualified personal trainer, see the following sidebar.

Selecting a Personal Trainer

A personal trainer should meet certain qualifications. The title of "personal trainer" does not tell you if the person has the necessary background; unfortunately selecting a trainer is truly a "buyer beware" situation because there are no mandated standards on what qualifications are needed to be a personal trainer. You will need to ask some specific questions to determine if the person has the appropriate qualifications. When meeting with a potential trainer, cover this list of questions, and look for a different trainer if you find many of the answers to be no.

1. Does the trainer have a college degree in a health and fitness field? (Look for degree names such as exercise science, physical education, or kinesiology.)

2. Does the trainer hold a nationally recognized certification from a not-for-profit organization? You can look for ACSM-certified professionals in your area by using ACSM's Pro Finder (see www.acsm.org). Other organizations also provide solid certifications, including the National Strength and Conditioning Association.

3. Is the trainer involved in continuing education opportunities to remain current?

4. Is the trainer certified in CPR and first aid?

5. Does the trainer have liability insurance?

6. Does the trainer have sufficient experience working with older female clients?

(continued)

(continued)

7. Does the trainer use preactivity screenings and fitness assessments?
8. Did the trainer ask you about medications and your health history?
9. Will the sessions include cardiorespiratory, muscular, and flexibility training?
10. Are the session length and cost reasonable?

Selecting a qualified personal trainer will require you to interview the person. This list of questions is a starting point. You should also consider whether your personality matches that of the trainer. Do you feel at ease with the person? Do you feel the trainer really listens to you and can understand your goals? Hiring a trainer is not a necessity, but if you make the investment, be sure to find out his or her educational background and certifications.

Stay-at-Home Options

A health club or the local YMCA may not always be the best fit for everyone, and there are times when traveling to a facility is inconvenient. Fortunately, numerous options are available for home exercise. Many cardiorespiratory conditioning activities do not require much equipment. For example, if you want to walk or jog, you can easily head out the front door. When using roads or sidewalks, remember safety tips. Always face traffic, and stay in safe, familiar areas. Wearing a headset is not recommended because you should be constantly aware of your surroundings.

If you are not comfortable with outdoor activities, you may want to purchase exercise equipment for home use. One former student shared her choice to purchase a treadmill. As a gift from her husband she was given the option of a yearly health club membership or a treadmill. She chose the treadmill. Although the cost was obviously much higher than a single year's membership, over the years she has saved club membership costs, and the treadmill allows her to train on her own schedule. When I called her home one afternoon, her teenage daughter said, "Mom is exercising and will call you back in a couple of hours." Thinking this was a misstatement proved incorrect. "Mom" was in training for a marathon and was completing a two-hour run on her treadmill!

As noted in chapter 4, you can include muscular strength and endurance training at home. Using your own body weight with sit-ups, push-ups, and pull-ups is the least expensive option. For minimal cost you can purchase dumbbells or elastic bands to provide resistance. As with cardiorespiratory conditioning, home-based resistance equipment may also be attractive.

The market for home exercise equipment has greatly expanded in the past 10 years. The people selling equipment on the infomercials look so happy and so fit, how could you go wrong? Unfortunately, making the wrong selection may result in wasted money as well as frustration. What should you consider when buying home exercise equipment? The following is a list of questions to ask yourself before you buy:

• What are my fitness goals? If your goal is to walk 30 minutes four days per week, then you do not need to purchase a treadmill with a capability to train an Olympic marathoner. On the other hand, if you desire to improve to the point of competitive running in local races, then you will want a treadmill that can handle the rigors of your training. The concept of matching your use with the construction and purpose of the equipment is often overlooked.

• How much space do I have available? Take the time to measure the floor space available. When you look at an item on a showroom floor, it can appear small. But when it's in your spare bedroom, it may seem huge. You'll need some space around the equipment, so add several extra feet as you determine your space requirements. Also, consider ceiling height. Some resistance training equipment has a significant vertical component, so know how much height the room can accommodate.

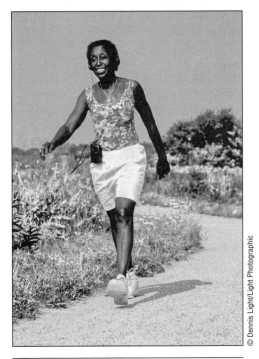

© Dennis Light/Light Photographic

• How much money do I want to spend? Home exercise equipment varies greatly in price. When you're considering cost, obviously your budget plays a central role. You'll also want to reflect on the first question. If a simple piece of equipment will fulfill your purpose, then why purchase a more expensive piece of equipment with unnecessary options? Quality is another factor. Although your budget may be limited, an inexpensive piece of equipment that is poorly made will be a disappointing purchase. To ensure the quality will allow you years of enjoyable use, be selective in the number of items you purchase. Determining quality can be difficult, but examining all movable parts is a first step. Is the movement of the equipment

Through a healthy lifestyle and a well-planned exercise program, don't just survive menopause—thrive with it!

smooth or jerky? Smooth, fluid motion of movable parts is a sign of good workmanship. Does the equipment come with a warranty? How long has the item been in production? Warranties and longevity do not guarantee quality but are considerations.

• How does the equipment feel? Never purchase a piece of equipment you cannot try. It is unlikely you would purchase a vehicle only by looking at a picture in a magazine. Similarly, you should try the item (or a showroom model of that particular item) before purchasing. We recommend going to a showroom floor dressed to exercise. When one of the authors purchased a treadmill for home use, she arrived at the showroom, asked the salesperson for permission, and then proceeded to run on one treadmill after another after another, returning to the top two choices before making a final selection. Each brand and model (whether a treadmill, a bike, or a resistance training machine or frame) will have a different fit and feel. Taking the time to "test-drive" the equipment will help you avoid disappointment when you take it home. Any piece of equipment you cannot try, you likely should not buy.

• Is assembly provided? Once a selection is made, you will receive a box with your equipment "to be assembled." For some items, this may be simple, but for others assembly may be difficult or nearly impossible. If you do not have someone to assist you, or are not mechanically inclined, discuss options available for delivery and assembly of the equipment with the salesperson.

Some of the most common pieces of home exercise equipment are treadmills, stationary bikes, and resistance training equipment. Specific recommendations for each are in the sidebar on this page.

Flexibility exercises are the simplest activities to include in a home-based program. Equipment is not necessary, and you may include stretching activities in your overall wind-down from the day. You could purchase a mat for comfort, but a towel on a carpeted floor can serve the same purpose.

Exercise videotapes focusing on flexibility, strength, and cardiorespiratory fitness are available. It is beyond the scope of this book to evaluate the myriad videos currently on the market. Consider the credentials of the person producing the tape, and only do those activities within your current fitness abilities. When trying a new workout, do not go 100 percent the first time because new exercise may lead to soreness for a few days. Start slowly and gradually, always evaluating the appropriateness of the workouts.

Selecting Home Exercise Equipment

Selecting a piece of exercise equipment is an important decision—both in terms of function as well as finance. Here is some information on three of the more commonly purchased items: treadmills, stationary bikes, and resistance training equipment.

TREADMILLS

In general, a motor-driven treadmill is recommended. We recommend at least a 2.5 horsepower motor, especially if you plan to jog or run on the treadmill. Some treadmills require a 110-volt electrical outlet, while others require 220 volts. Be sure that your home can accommodate the power supply requirements. In addition to the motor, examine the belt and the bed the belt moves over. The belt should be heavy duty to prevent it from stretching excessively over time. There should be no hesitation of the belt with each foot strike. Just like an automobile, each treadmill has a different feel or ride. Some treadmills have a softer, more cushioned feel, which many walkers enjoy. Other treadmills have a firmer, more rigid feel, which may be better for joggers or runners. The treadmill should never feel wobbly—even when on an incline.

Available treadmill display options seem endless. Baseline information should include time, speed, and grade (incline). The range of speed and grade options will depend on your overall goals. When testing the treadmill at the showroom, exercise at the speed and grade you plan to use in training. Does the treadmill move easily from one speed to another? Does the treadmill incline and decline smoothly? If the answer to either question is no, then try another treadmill. Other optional features to consider include side handrails, heart rate monitoring capabilities, and custom programming of workouts. All treadmills should have an emergency shutoff feature.

Although not part of the treadmill, a good pair of walking or running shoes will definitely influence your enjoyment of the treadmill. Look for a pair of shoes with good support and cushioning that fit your feet properly. When walking or jogging on a treadmill, keep your eyes focused out in front of you rather than down at your feet (which may make you feel dizzy) or out to the side (which may cause you to drift off the belt).

STATIONARY BIKES

Stationary bikes are great pieces of home exercise equipment because of their relatively small size and low price. Both upright and semirecumbent models use some type of resistance on the flywheel to increase and decrease the workload. Some bikes use suspended weights and friction belts, some use magnetic resistance or hydraulics, and others use air. The ability to adjust the bike to your body size is important. Check that the seat height and handlebar positions can be adjusted to your comfort (your knees should have a slight bend when at the bottom of the pedal stroke, and the handlebars should not cause you to reach extensively or feel restricted). The seat should feel comfortable to you and should be adjusted to be relatively level (rather than pointing too far up or down). Spend some time adjusting the bike to a comfortable position. Pedaling should be smooth and fluid—not halting at the top or bottom of the pedal stroke. There are benefits to pedals with straps (allowing you to both push down and pull up with each revolution), so consider that option as well.

(continued)

(continued)

The extent of the digital display will depend on your preference. Realize that most calorie counters provide only ballpark estimates of calories expended. At a minimum, a display should show the resistance level and time. Some bikes require electricity, so keep appropriate voltage availability in mind when selecting a model.

RESISTANCE TRAINING EQUIPMENT

Resistance training equipment includes a range of items, from simple dumbbells to large multistation machines with weight plates and pulleys. If you desire overall muscular strength and endurance conditioning at home, you can purchase ankle weights and a set of dumbbells of various weights. Pay attention to the quality of the weights, and make sure you have a good place to store them (a weight rack can be helpful if space is limited). In addition, purchasing elastic bands of various levels of resistance will allow you to target almost all body parts.

Weightlifting frames allow you to perform barbell-related exercises. Multistation machines typically rely on weight stacks or hydraulic pistons to provide resistance for different exercises, with small changes needed in the machine configuration. When purchasing frames or other multistation resistance machines, consider the overall construction. Is the base sufficiently wide to prevent turnover of the equipment? Are the joint connections sufficiently stable and sturdy? Each piece of resistance training equipment must meet a certain level of quality to allow for safe use. Depending on the equipment, you may need to determine if your floor can handle the weight as well as the overall size of the unit (length, width, and height). Check that you can adjust the equipment for your limb and body size. Equipment manufacturers focus more on men, so the adjustments do not always accommodate the smaller size of women.

Finding the Balance

A balanced exercise program is the focus of this book. Some changes occurring in your body are due to menopause and some are due to the aging process in general. As emphasized in chapter 2, a complete exercise program involves three components: cardiorespiratory endurance, muscular strength and endurance, and flexibility. Each component is beneficial to you as a woman.

You should work on cardiorespiratory endurance three to five days per week. The selection of activity will vary depending on your interest and what is available. The benefits of a regular exercise program cannot be overemphasized. Completing a fitness assessment as described in chapter 3 is helpful when starting your program; you should complete an assessment every three or four months so you can reevaluate your status.

Muscular strength and endurance are so important for women—especially as they age. Incorporate resistance training into your plan at least two days per week. The use of dumbbells, weight machines, or elastic resistance bands all can provide the necessary overload on your muscles for improvements in your muscular fitness. As with your cardiorespiratory fitness, repeating the assessments of muscular strength and endurance described in chapter 4 can be helpful in charting your progress.

Flexibility is an often neglected part of an exercise program. The benefits to be gained from good flexibility are outlined in chapter 5. Use of the assessment tools periodically can, once again, provide feedback on gains in flexibility as a result of a regular stretching regimen.

The New You

Perimenopause and postmenopause are times in a woman's life filled with changes and challenges. Some of these are related to hormonal and associated physiological changes, which may present challenges to keeping a "life as normal" perspective. We suggest you forget the search for "normal" because we have found it to be an elusive goal and impossible to define (other than a hopeful dream or a rosy view of the past). Rather, each day is filled not only with changes and challenges but also with new opportunities. We hope that one of those new opportunities is your exercise program. Carpe diem—seize the day!

ACTION PLAN:
MAINTAINING YOUR MOTIVATION

- ☐ Keep an activity log for your cardiorespiratory, muscular, and flexibility training.
- ☐ Develop your own personalized adherence pledge.
- ☐ Reevaluate your progress monthly, and update your short-term goals.
- ☐ Determine what type of program best fits into your schedule (organized program, health club, home-based program):
  - If joining a health club, select one carefully using the list of questions given in this chapter.
  - If using a home-based program, consider what equipment you may want to purchase using the buyer's guide presented in this chapter.

RESOURCES

Many resources are available for additional information regarding menopause. For books, videos, and CDs, check with your local public library. If the materials you seek are not available, check with a librarian to determine if the item can be borrowed from another library (often called interlibrary loan). Use the Internet to obtain the latest information from the Web sites of national organizations such as the North American Menopause Society and the American College of Obstetricians and Gynecologists. Your gynecologist and local medical centers are other good resources to utilize. Ask for a schedule of upcoming presentations or seminars regarding menopause, exercise, and other women's health issues.

Hormone therapy is a hot area of research, with new results from studies being released frequently. Know your medical history and the contraindications for hormone therapy, and maintain open communication with your physician or gynecologist. Study the latest and sometimes conflicting reports carefully, and weigh the choices before making decisions. Be certain the reports you read have been written by qualified health professionals or released by a respected health organization or institution.

As you develop your action plan for personal fitness, use local resources for motivation. Radio, television, and newspapers provide updates on upcoming fitness events (e.g., walks, 5K runs, bike-a-thons, master's swimming events) and present regular health-related news features. Evaluate the options at local fitness centers, both private and public, and determine what facilities and equipment (e.g., swimming pools, track, weight equipment) are available to the public at local schools and universities. Talk to friends about where they exercise and in what activities they participate.

The variety of resources in the following list offers a wide range of reliable information concerning your personal health, fitness, and menopause questions. The American College of Sports Medicine provides the standard for exercise guidelines and safety. Other organizations and agencies present the latest information regarding nutrition, aging, and women's health. Carefully assess the reliability of all health-related information.

Organizations and Agencies

American Cancer Society (information on cancer prevention and treatment)
Public Information Department
1599 Clifton Road, NE
Atlanta, GA 30329
1-800-ACS-2345
www.cancer.org

American College of Obstetricians and Gynecologists (information on
hormone therapy, menopause-related health issues, and locating a
board-certified gynecologist under Find a Physician)
409 12th St., SW
P.O. Box 96920
Washington, DC 20090-6920
www.acog.org

American College of Sports Medicine (fitness information and how to find
an ACSM-certified exercise professional in your community)
401 W. Michigan St.
Indianapolis, IN 46202-3233
317-673-9200
www.acsm.org

American Diabetes Association (nutrition and diabetes information)
1701 North Beauregard Street
Alexandria, VA 22311
1-800-DIABETES (1-800-342-2383)
www.diabetes.org

American Dietetic Association (nutrition information and also the Women's
Bone Health Quiz found under the Food and Nutrition Information link)
216 W. Jackson Boulevard
Suite 800
Chicago, IL 60606-6995
1-800-366-1655
www.eatright.org

American Heart Association (nutrition and heart health information)
7272 Greenville Avenue
Dallas, TX 75231-4596
1-800-242-8721
www.americanheart.org
www.justmove.org/home.cfm (has a good activity guide to set goals and to
track progress)

American Medical Association (medical information on many topics, including women's health)
515 North State Street
Chicago, IL 60610
1-800-621-8335
www.ama-assn.org

American Menopause Foundation (menopause research, literature, and information)
350 Fifth Avenue
Suite 2822
New York, NY 10118
212-714-2398
www.americanmenopause.org

Centers for Disease Control and Prevention (information on disease prevention and health promotion)
National Center for Chronic Disease Prevention and Health Promotion
Division of Nutrition and Physical Activity, MS K-46
4770 Buford Highway, NE
Atlanta, Georgia 30341-3724
1-888-CDC-4NRG (1-888-232-4674)
www.cdc.gov

Food and Drug Administration (drug and hormone therapy information)
5600 Fishers Lane
Rockville MD 20857-0001
1-888-INFO-FDA (1-888-463-6332)
www.fda.gov/womens/menopause

International Menopause Society (the official voice of the affiliated menopause societies)
Jean Wright, IMS Executive Director
P.O. Box 687, Wray
Lancaster LA2 8WY, UK
+44 15242 21190
jwright.ims@btopenworld.com
www.imsociety.org

National Association for Health and Fitness (health and fitness information)
201 South Capitol Avenue
Suite 560
Indianapolis, IN 46225
317-237-5360
www.physicalfitness.org

National Heart, Lung, and Blood Institute (see information on the Women's Health Initiative, WHI, by going to the Web site and then entering Women's Health Initiative or menopause in the search box)
P.O. Box 30105
Bethesda, MD 20824-0105
301-251-1222
www.nhlbi.nih.gov

National Institute on Aging Information Center (healthy aging information)
P.O. Box 8057
Gaithersburg, MD 20898-8057
1-800-222-2225
www.nia.nih.gov

National Institutes of Health (wide variety of health-related information)
9000 Rockville Pike
Bethesda, MD 20892
301-496-4461
www.nih.gov

National Osteoporosis Foundation (comprehensive resource on bone health and osteoporosis)
1150 17th St., NW
Suite 500
Washington, DC 20036-4603
202-223-2226
www.nof.org

National Strength and Conditioning Association (resistance training information)
P.O. Box 38909
Colorado Springs, CO 80937-8909
719-632-6722
www. nsca-lift.org

National Women's Health Resource Center (national clearinghouse for women's health information)
157 Broad Street
Suite 315
Red Bank, NJ 07701
1-877-986-9472
www.healthywomen.org

North American Menopause Society (NAMS) (information on menopause along with resources such as the *Menopause Guidebook*)
P.O. Box 94527
Cleveland, OH 44101
440-442-7550
info@menopause.org
www.menopause.org

U.S. Department of Agriculture (nutrition information)
Food and Nutrition Information Center
10301 Baltimore Boulevard
Room 304
Beltsville, MD 20705-2351
301-504-5719
fnic@nal.usda.gov

U.S. Department of Health and Human Services (includes women's health and menopause information)
Public Health Service, National Institutes of Health
200 Independence Avenue, SW
Washington, DC 20201
1-877-696-6775
www.hhs.gov

Additional Web Sites

Agency for Healthcare Research and Quality (information on the quality, safety, and effectiveness of health care)
www.ahrq.gov
See the Prevention and Wellness link (www.ahrq.gov/consumer/index.html#prevention) to find the *Pocket Guide to Staying Healthy at 50+* (a comprehensive booklet with tips on good health habits, screening tests, and immunizations for older Americans).

Dietary Guidelines for Americans (resource for the latest recommendations on intakes of nutrients)
www.healthierus.gov/dietaryguidelines

Gatorade Sports Science Institute (resource for research in the area of sports and nutrition)
www.gssiweb.com

Mayo Clinic (health, fitness, and menopause information)
www.mayoclinic.com

Medem Network (online consultation and medical library)
www.Medem.com

MEDSCAPE from WebMD (medical information on a wide variety of topics)
www.medscape.com/homepage

National Women's Health Information Center (a division of US DHHS,
   Office on Women's Health; provides information on hormone therapy
   and menopause)
1-800-994-WOMAN (1-800-994-9662)
www.4woman.gov/Menopause

Sources of information on MET values on the Internet:
   www.plu.edu/~chasega/met.html
   prevention.sph.sc.edu/tools/compendium.htm

Books

Action Plan for Arthritis, by A. Lynn Millar, 2003, Human Kinetics
   (source for exercise plans for those with arthritis)

Full-Body Flexibility, by Jay Blahnik, 2004, Human Kinetics (source for
   many different stretching exercises)

Nancy Clark's Sports Nutrition Guidebook, Third Edition, by Nancy
   Clark, 2003, Human Kinetics (down-to-earth information,
   including simple recipes, on eating to fuel an active lifestyle)

Nutrition for Health, Fitness & Sport, Sixth Edition, by Melvin
   H. Williams, 2002, McGraw-Hill (great source for calorie
   value information on a wide variety of activities, as well as
   comprehensive information on nutrition)

Strength Training Past 50, by Wayne L. Westcott and Thomas R.
   Baechle, 1998, Human Kinetics (source for many different
   resistance training exercises)

GLOSSARY

adherence—The ability to continue or maintain an exercise program.

aerobic—Means "with oxygen"; often used with regard to endurance-type exercise.

aerobic exercise—Includes activities that use large muscle groups in a repetitive fashion, thus increasing heart rate and respiration rate.

atherosclerosis—A thickening or hardening of the interior lining of the artery walls caused by plaque (fatty substances) deposits, resulting in a narrowing of arteries.

atrophy—Decreasing muscle size; usually due to injury, inactivity, or illness.

ballistic stretch—A sudden bouncing stretch that can result in torn muscles and tendons.

body mass index (BMI)—A number used to assess weight relative to height; involves dividing body weight expressed in kilograms (convert from pounds by dividing by 2.2) by the square of body height expressed in meters (convert from inches by multiplying by 0.0254); units are kg/m^2.

bone mineral density (BMD) tests—A low-dose X ray of bone to screen for osteoporosis.

cardiorespiratory endurance (aka cardiorespiratory fitness)—The ability of the body to perform large muscle, dynamic, moderate- to high-intensity exercise for prolonged time periods.

carotid pulse—Heart rate determined by placing gentle pressure on the side of the neck next to the windpipe where the carotid artery lies close to the skin.

cholesterol ratio—A ratio calculated by dividing the total cholesterol level by the HDL cholesterol level.

concentric muscle contraction—Contraction when the muscles shorten to move or lift an object.

contraindication—Reasons not to use a product or to do an activity.

cortical bone (aka compact bone)—Dense, hard bone that forms the external layer of bones.

diastolic pressure—The amount of pressure on the arteries when the heart is between beats or at rest; lower number of a blood pressure reading.

double progressive program—Used in weight training to increase the repetitions and then the resistance.

dual energy X-ray absorptiometry (DEXA)—The most accurate test of bone mineral density (BMD) currently available.

duration—How long a person exercises during one session.

dyslipidemia—Abnormal blood levels of cholesterol and triglycerides.

dyspareunia—Painful intercourse.

eccentric muscle contraction—Contraction when the muscles lengthen during controlled lowering of an object or weight.

estrogen—Female hormone responsible for changes in female sexual characteristics at puberty; also related to bone health, it occurs in various forms (estriol, estrone, and estradiol).

estrone—The main type of estrogen remaining after menopause; a weaker form of estrogen than estradiol, estrone is produced within fat tissue.

exercise progression—See overload or principle of progression.

extensibility (aka "stretchability")—The ability of the muscles to stretch.

flexibility—When a single joint or multiple joints can move freely through full movement or range of motion to perform specific tasks.

flexion (aka bending)—When movement at a joint causes two body parts to move toward one another.

follicle-stimulating hormone (FSH)—A female hormone that stimulates the growth of a group of cells (follicle) that surround a developing egg.

frequency—How often a person exercises each week.

HDL (high-density lipoprotein) cholesterol—Protein–lipid complex that moves excess cholesterol out of the arteries, thereby protecting against cardiovascular diseases ("good" cholesterol).

heart rate monitor—A simple device (a special strap worn around the torso) that transmits electrical information from the heart to a receiver, allowing for a display of heart rate.

homocysteine—An amino acid found in the body that is thought to damage the lining of arteries and thus is associated with increased risk of heart disease.

hormone therapy (HT) (previously known as hormone replacement therapy, HRT)—The prescription use of estrogen or estrogen and progestin in perimenopausal women to reduce the symptoms caused by hot flashes, vaginal atrophy, and postmenopausal osteoporosis.

hot flash—A feeling of heat in the upper part of a woman's body (face, neck, and upper torso) or bodywide, often accompanied by perspiration and red blotching of the skin; hot flashes occurring during sleep are termed "night sweats."

hypertrophy—Muscle growth by increases in the size of muscle cells.

hypothalamus—The control center of the brain that signals the pituitary and the ovaries to release female hormones each month to create the menstrual cycle.

intensity—How hard a person exercises.

isokinetic—A type of weight machine that utilizes constant speed and resistance throughout the range of motion.

isometric (aka static) **muscle contraction**—Contraction without movement or change in muscle length.

isotonic (aka dynamic) **muscle contraction**—Contraction with a change in length of the muscle; may involve push-ups, weight machines, or free weights.

LDL (low-density lipoprotein) cholesterol—Protein–lipid complex that transports cholesterol to the organs and tissues; high levels are associated with increased risk of coronary heart disease ("bad" cholesterol).

longitudinal studies—Research studies continually examining a group of people, conducted over an extended time period.

luteinizing hormone (LH)—A female hormone that signals the ovaries to release the egg so ovulation occurs.

maximal heart rate—Highest heart rate possible during a maximal exercise test; also commonly estimated by subtracting a person's age from 220.

menarche—The first menstrual cycle; typically occurs at the age of 12 or 13.

menopause—The cessation of menstruation, or the last menstrual period.

menses—The monthly flow of bloody fluid from the uterus; also known as a woman's monthly period.

MET (aka metabolic equivalent)—A term for the oxygen requirement of the body at rest.

metabolic rate—The rate the body burns calories (at rest and during activities).

monounsaturated fat—Fat that has a single double bond; found in canola, olive, and peanut oils.

muscular endurance—The ability of a muscle to make repeated contractions or to sustain a contraction.

muscular fitness—A general term that incorporates both muscular strength and muscular endurance.

muscular strength—The force the muscle can generate in one maximal effort.

nutrient density—The amount of nutrients per calorie in a given food.

nutrient-dense food—A food that contains the most nutrients with the least amount of calories.

one-repetition maximum (1RM) test—Test used to determine the greatest amount of weight that can be lifted one time for a given exercise.

opposing muscles—The muscles on the opposite side of the joint that have opposite functions.

osteoblasts—Cells that form new bone.

osteoclasts—Cells that break down bone.

osteopenia—Decreased bone density; often a precursor to osteoporosis.

osteoporosis—A type of skeletal deterioration or decreasing bone density that weakens the bone structure.

overload—Any activity beyond the normal level of exertion of that muscle or of that body system.

overtraining—Doing too much physical activity or exercise, which can cause unnecessary muscular soreness, fatigue, pain, or injury.

Pap tests—A scraping of cervical cells that are examined under a microscope as a screening test for cervical cancer.

perimenopause (aka climacteric or menopausal transition)—The time leading up to the last menstrual period and the following 12 months; a time of physical and hormonal changes.

physical fitness—The ability to perform physical activity; components of physical fitness are cardiovascular endurance, muscular strength and endurance, and flexibility.

pituitary—An endocrine gland that signals the release of hormones for the regulation of puberty, menstruation, growth, and other body functions.

placebo—A pill or medicine that resembles the real one but contains no active ingredients.

polyunsaturated fat—Fat that contains two or more double bonds; plant fat found in soybean, corn, sunflower, and safflower oils.

postmenopause—The time period beginning 12 months following the last menstrual cycle.

premenopause—The time of puberty until menopause; during this time, menstruation occurs approximately every 28 days.

principle of progression—Periodically increasing the amount or intensity of the workload (once the body adapts to it) in order to continue progress.

principle of specificity—The physical effects of exercise are specific to the muscles used and the activity or exercise performed.

progesterone—A female hormone produced by the ovaries; important for regulating the menstrual cycle as well as in preparing the uterus for a fertilized egg.

progressive resistance training (PRT)—A weight training program that places increasingly greater demands on the skeletal muscles.

proprioceptive neuromuscular facilitation (PNF)—A stretching technique in which the muscle is first contracted against a resistance and then is relaxed and stretched; usually requires a partner's assistance.

quantitative computerized tomography (QCT)—Low-dose X ray that produces a three-dimensional image of the spine.

radial pulse—Heart rate determined by placing gentle pressure on the inside of the wrist (thumb side) where the radial artery lies close to the skin.

range of motion—The amount a joint can be moved safely.

rating of perceived exertion (RPE)—A numerical ranking used to subjectively rank one's bodywide feeling of exertion during exercise; commonly used to guide exercise intensity.

repetition (aka "rep")—Lifting a weight one time.

resting metabolic rate—The amount of energy a person's body uses when under resting, nondigesting (postabsorptive) conditions.

reversibility—Concept that benefits are lost when training ceases.

risk factors—Characteristics associated with higher risk of a particular disease.

saturated fat—Fat with all carbon bonds filled; animal fats and coconut, palm, and palm kernel fats; contributes to increased blood cholesterol levels and cardiovascular diseases.

selective estrogen receptor modulators (SERMs)—Compounds that have some of the positive effects of estrogen (such as bone health) without other negative effects of estrogen (such as breast cancer).

set—Lifting a weight multiple times in succession; group of repetitions.

static stretch—A gentle, slow stretch or lengthening of the muscle(s) that is held for 10 to 30 seconds.

strength training (aka strength conditioning, weight training, resistance training)—A set of exercises that use the muscles against some external load.

stretching—Moving the joint, ligaments, muscles, and tendons through their ordinary range of motion and slightly beyond to generate slight muscle tension.

systolic pressure—A measure of the pressure on the arteries when the heart contracts; upper number of a blood pressure reading.

T-scores—A standardized score for bone density tests.

target exercise heart rate—The range of desired heart rate during aerobic exercise; typically 70 to 85 percent of maximal heart rate.

thermic effect of food—Energy requirement to digest, absorb, utilize, and store food that has been eaten.

trabecular bone (aka "spongy bone")—Bone with an open lattice-type structure; more affected than cortical (compact) bone by osteoporosis.

trans fatty acids (aka trans fats)—Fatty acids in which the hydrogen bonds are shifted to opposite sides of the double bond by a chemical process; found in processed (hydrogenated) vegetable fats and margarine; similar effects on the body as saturated fats.

triglycerides—A glycerol molecule with three fatty acid chains attached to it; main form in which fats are eaten and stored in the body; high levels may have a relationship with coronary artery disease.

$\dot{V}O_2$max—A measure of the maximum amount of oxygen the body can take in and use during maximal exercise; reflects cardiorespiratory fitness.

$\dot{V}O_2$max test—Laboratory test involving breathing through a mouthpiece and analysis of the oxygen consumed for determination of cardiorespiratory fitness.

weight-bearing exercise—Any activity in which a person bears her body weight; examples include walking and jogging.

REFERENCES

American Cancer Society. 2004. Can colorectal cancer and polyps be found early? [Online]. Available: www.cancer.org [October 4, 2004].

———. 2003. Answers to questions often asked by cancer survivors about nutrition and physical activity. *Cancer Journal for Clinicians* 53: 303-309.

American College of Obstetricians and Gynecologists (ACOG). 2003a. Making lovemaking last. *American College of Obstetricians and Gynecologists' Guide to Managing Menopause and the Years Beyond* (7)2: 42-44.

———. 2003b. Your changing health care needs. *American College of Obstetricians and Gynecologists' Guide to Managing Menopause and the Years Beyond* (7)2: 8.

———. 2003c. The change: How menopause affects you. *American College of Obstetricians and Gynecologists' Guide to Managing Menopause and the Years Beyond* (7)2: 10-12.

———. 2003d. Bones that last a lifetime. *American College of Obstetricians and Gynecologists' Guide to Managing Menopause and the Years Beyond.* (7)2: 43-44.

———. 2002. Questions and answers on hormone therapy. [Online]. Available: www.medem.com [June 14, 2004].

American College of Sports Medicine (ACSM). 2005. *ACSM's guidelines for exercise testing and prescription.* 7th ed. Baltimore: Lippincott Williams & Wilkins.

———. 2004. Position stand: Physical activity and bone health. *Medicine & Science in Sports & Exercise* 36(11): 1985-1996.

———. 2003a. *ACSM fitness book.* 3rd ed. Champaign, IL: Human Kinetics.

———. 2003b. Five easy steps to beginning strength exercises. ACSM's Active Aging Partnership and the Strategic Health Initiative on Aging. [Online]. Available: www.acsm.org/health%2Bfitness/activeaging.htm [June 19, 2004].

———. 2002. Position stand: Progression models in resistance training for healthy adults. *Medicine & Science in Sports & Exercise* 34(2): 364-380.

———. 2001. *ACSM's resource manual for guidelines for exercise testing and prescription.* 4th ed. Baltimore: Williams & Wilkins.

———. 2000. *ACSM's guidelines for exercise testing and prescription.* 6th ed. Baltimore: Lippincott Williams & Wilkins.

———. 1999. Exercise your way to lower blood pressure. [Online]. Available: www.acsm.org/pdf/Hypert.pdf [June 19, 2004].

———. 1998a. Position stand: Exercise and physical activity for older adults. *Medicine & Science in Sports & Exercise* 30(6): 992-1008.

———. 1998b. Position stand: The recommended quantity and quality of exercise for developing and maintaining cardiorespiratory and muscular fitness, and flexibility in healthy adults. *Medicine & Science in Sports & Exercise* 30(6): 975-991.

———. 1998c. *ACSM's resource manual for guidelines for exercise testing and prescription.* 3rd ed. Baltimore: Williams & Wilkins.

————. 1995. Position stand: Osteoporosis and exercise. *Medicine & Science in Sports & Exercise* 27(4): i-vii.

American Dietetic Association (ADA). 2004. Position of the American Dietetic Association and Dietitians of Canada: Nutrition and women's health. *Journal of the American Dietetic Association* (104)7: 984-1001.

————. 2002a. Position of the American Dietetic Association: Health implications of dietary fiber. *Journal of the American Dietetic Association* (102)7: 993-1000.

————. 2002b. Total diet approach to communicating food and nutrition information. *Journal of the American Dietetic Association* 102: 100. [Online]. Available: www.eatright.org.Public/GovernmentAffairs/92_adar_0102.cfm [June 19, 2004].

————. 2000. Speak up for five a day. American Dietetic Association fact sheet. [Online]. Available: www.eatright.org/Public/NutritionInformation/92_nfs0700.cfm [June 19, 2004].

American Heart Association (AHA). 2004. What are healthy levels of cholesterol? [Online]. Available: www.americanheart.org/presenter.jhtml?identifier=183 [June 19, 2004].

American Thyroid Association (ATA). 2004. 2004 thyroid awareness campaign encourages patients and physicians to take control of thyroid health. [Online]. Available: www.thyroid.org/professionals/publications/news/04_01_21_awareness_campaign.html [July 6, 2004].

Ash, D., and C.J. Werlinger. 1997. *Exercises for health promotion.* Gaithersburg, MD: Aspen.

Baechle, T.R., and R.W. Earle. 1995. *Fitness weight training.* Champaign, IL: Human Kinetics.

Ballard, K. 2003. *Understanding menopause.* West Sussex: Wiley.

Banks, E., V. Beral, G. Reeves, A. Balkwill, and I. Barnes. 2004. Fracture incidence in relation to the pattern of use of hormone therapy in postmenopausal women. *Journal of the American Medical Association* 291(18): 2212-2220.

Bassey, E.J., M.J. Bendall, and M. Pearson. 1988. Muscle strength in the triceps surae and objectively measured customary walking activity in men and women over 65 years of age. *Clinical Science* 74: 85-89.

Beach, F.A. 1976. Sexual attractivity, proceptivity, and receptivity in female mammals. *Hormonal Behavior* 7: 105-138.

Beaulieu, J.E. 1980. *Stretching for all sports.* Pasadena, CA: Athletic.

Best Clinical Practices. 2002. International Position Paper on Women's Health and Menopause: A Comprehensive Approach. National Heart, Lung and Blood Institute; Office of Research on Women's Health; National Institutes of Health; and Giovanni Lorenzini Medical Science Foundation.

Blahnik, J. 2004. *Full-body flexibility.* Champaign, IL: Human Kinetics.

Bone density testing: Measure your risk of broken bones. 2004. [Online]. Available: mayoclinic.com/printinvoker.cfm?objected=302A6991-185F-4E75-B6399FED [May 19, 2004].

Boyle, M.A., and G. Zyla. 1996. *Personal nutrition.* 3rd ed. Minneapolis: West.

Brown, J.K., T. Byers, C. Doyle, K.S. Coumeya, W. Demark-Wahnefried, L.H. Kushi, A. Mc-Tieman, C.L. Rock, J. Aziz, A.B. Bloch, B. Eldridge, K. Hamilton, C. Katzin, A. Koonce, J. Main, C. Mobley, M.E. Morra, M.S. Pierce, and K.A. Sawyer. 2003. Nutritional and physical activity during and after cancer treatment: An American Cancer Society guide for informed choices. *Cancer Journal for Clinicians* 53: 268-291.

Brubaker, P., L. Kaminsky, and M. Whaley. 2002. *Coronary artery disease: Essentials of prevention and rehabilitation programs.* Champaign, IL: Human Kinetics.

Burghardt, M. 1999. Exercise at menopause: A critical difference. *Medscape General Medicine* 1(3). [Online]. Available: www.medscape.com/viewarticle/408896 [October 28, 2003].

Byers, T., M. Nestle, A. McTiernan, C. Doyle, A. Currie-Williams, T. Gansler, and M. Thun. 2002. American Cancer Society 2001 Nutrition and Physical Activity Guidelines Advisory Committee. American Cancer Society guidelines on nutrition and physical activity for cancer prevention: Reducing the risk of cancer with healthy food choices and physical activity. *Cancer Journal for Clinicians* 52: 92-119.

Canadian Society for Exercise Physiology (CESP). 2003. *The Canadian physical activity, fitness & lifestyle approach: CSEP-health & fitness program's health-related appraisal and counselling strategy.* 3rd ed. Ottawa, Canada. 7-37 to7-52.

Cauley, J.A., J. Robbins, Z. Chen, S.R. Cummings, R.D. Jackson, A.Z. LaCroix, M. LeBoff, C.E. Lewis, J. McGowan, J. Neuner, M. Pettinger, M.L. Stefanick, J. Wactawski-Wende, and N.B. Watts. 2003. Effects of estrogen plus progestin on risk of fractures and bone mineral density: The Women's Health Initiative randomized trial. *Journal of the American Medical Association* 290(13): 1729-1738.

Chlebowski, R.T., S.L. Hendrix, R.D. Langer, M.L. Stefanick, M. Gass, D. Lane, R.J. Rodabough, M.A. Gilligan, M.G. Cyr, C.A. Thomson, J. Khandekar, H. Petrovitch, and A. McTiernan. 2003. Influence of estrogen plus progestin on breast cancer and mammography in healthy postmenopausal women: The Women's Health Initiative randomized trial. *Journal of the American Medical Association* 289(24): 3243-3253.

Chlebowski, R.T., J. Wactawski-Wende, C. Ritenbaugh, A. Hubbell, J. Ascensao, R.J. Rodabough, C.A. Rosenberg, V.M. Taylor, R. Harris, C. Chen, L.L. Adams-Campbell, and E. White. 2004. Estrogen plus progestin and colorectal cancer in postmenopausal women. *New England Journal of Medicine* 350(10): 991-1004.

Cohn, S.H., D. Vartsky, S. Yasumura, A. Savitsky, I. Zanzi, A. Vaswani, and K.J. Ellis. 1980. Compartmental body composition based on total-body potassium and calcium. *American Journal of Physiology* 239: E534-E530.

Corbin, C.B., R. Lindsey, G.J. Welk, and W.R. Corbin. 2002. *Concepts of fitness and wellness.* 4th ed. New York: McGraw-Hill.

Current issues in flexibility fitness. June 2000. *President's Council on Physical Fitness and Sports Research Digest.* Series 3, Number 10. [Online]. Available: www.indiana.edu/~prechal [February 2, 2004].

Cussler, E., T.G. Lohman, S.B. Going, L.B. Houtkooper, L.L. Metcalfe, H.G. Flint-Wagner, R.B. Harris, and P.J. Teixeira. 2003. Weight lifted in strength training predicts bone change in postmenopausal women. *Medicine & Science in Sports & Exercise* 35(1): 10-17.

Delmas, P.D., N.H. Bjarnason, B.H. Mitlak, A.C. Ravoux, A.S. Shah, W.J. Huster, M. Draper, and C. Christiansen. 1997. Effects of Raloxifene on bone mineral density, serum cholesterol concentrations, and uterine endometrium in postmenopausal women. *New England Journal of Medicine* 337(23): 1641-1647.

deVries, H. 1981. Physiology of exercise. *Journal of Physical Education, Recreation & Dance* (52)41: 1980.

Dietary Guidelines for Americans (DGA). 2005a. Department of Health and Human Services and Department of Agriculture. [Online]. Available: www.healthierus.gov/dietaryguidelines [January 13, 2005].

Dietary Guidelines for Americans (DGA). 2005b. Department of Health and Human Services and Department of Agriculture. [Online]. Available: www.healthierus.gov/dietaryguidelines/dga2005/report [October 9, 2004].

Draper, M.W. 2003. The role of selective estrogen receptor modulators (SERMs) in postmenopausal health. In *Women's Health and Disease: Gynecologic and Reproductive*

Issues, ed. G. Creatsas, G. Mastorakos, and G.P. Chrousos, 373-377. New York: New York Academy of Sciences.

Drinkwater, B.L. 1999. Exercise and bone in the postmenopausal years: A reality check. In *The Menopause at the Millennium,* ed. T. Aso, T. Yanaihara, and S. Fujimoto, 212-215. New York: Parthenon.

Ebben, W.P., and R.L. Jensen. 1998. Strength training for women: Debunking myths that block opportunity. *Physician and Sportsmedicine.* 26(5). [Online]. Available: www.physsportsmed.com/issues/1998/05may/ebben.htm [February 19, 2004].

Evans, W.J., and W.W. Campbell. 1993. Sarcopenia and age-related changes in body composition and functional capacity. *Journal of Nutrition* 123: 465-68.

Fahey, T.D., P.M. Insel, and W.T. Roth. 2003. *Fit & Well.* 5th ed. New York: McGraw-Hill.

Fleck, S.J., and W.J. Kraemer. 1997. *Designing resistance training programs.* 2nd ed. Champaign, IL: Human Kinetics.

Franklin, B.A., and K. Chinnaiyan. 2004. New guidelines for cardiovascular disease prevention in women. *American Journal of Medicine & Sports* 6(2): 50-51.

Freedman, R.R., and W. Krell. 1999. Reduced thermoregulatory null zone in postmenopausal women with hot flashes. *American Journal of Obstetrics and Gynecology* 181(1): 66-70.

Freedman, R.R., and S. Woodward. 1992. Behavioral treatment of menopausal hot flushes: Evaluation by ambulatory monitoring. *American Journal of Obstetrics and Gynecology* 167(2): 436-439.

Freedman, R.R., S. Woodward, B. Brown, J.I. Javaid, and G.N. Pandey. 1995. Biochemical and thermoregulatory effects of behavioral treatment for menopausal hot flashes. *Menopause: The Journal of the North American Menopause Society* 2(4): 211-218.

Gann, P.H., and M. Morrow. 2003. Combined hormone therapy and breast cancer: A single-edged sword. *Journal of the American Medical Association* 289(24): 3304-3306.

Gold, E.B., B. Sternfeld, J.L. Kelsey, C. Brown, C. Mouton, N. Reame, L. Salamone, and R. Stellato. 2000. Relation of demographic and lifestyle factors to symptoms in a multiracial/ethnic population of women 40-55 years of age. *American Journal of Epidemiology* 152(5): 463-473.

Goldman, M.B., and M.C. Hatch, eds. 2000. *Women and health.* San Diego: Academic Press.

Graves, J.E., and B.A. Franklin, eds. 2001. *Resistance training for health and rehabilitation.* Champaign, IL: Human Kinetics.

Griffin, J.C. 1998. *Client-centered exercise prescription.* Champaign, IL: Human Kinetics.

Hales, D., and C. Zartman. 2001. *An invitation to fitness & wellness.* Belmont, CA: Wadsworth/Thomson Learning.

Hammar, M., G. Berg, and R. Lindgren. 1990. Does physical exercise influence the frequency of postmenopausal hot flushes? *Acta Obstetricia et Gynecologica Scandinavica* 69: 409-412.

Heyward, V.H. 2002. *Advanced fitness assessment and exercise prescription.* 4th ed. Champaign, IL: Human Kinetics.

Hoeger, W.K, and S.A. Hoeger. 2002. *Principles and labs for physical fitness.* 3rd ed. Belmont, CA: Wadsworth/Thomson Learning.

Holt, J., L.E. Holt, and T.W. Pellham. 1996. Flexibility redefined. In *Biomechanics in sports XIII,* ed. T. Bauer, 172. Thunder Bay, Ontario: Lakehead University.

Hopkins, P.N., and E.A. Brinton. 2003. Estrogen receptor 1 variants and coronary artery disease: Shedding light into a murky pool. *Journal of the American Medical Association* 290(17): 2317-2319.

Howley, E.T., and B.D. Franks. 2003. *Health fitness instructor's handbook.* 4th ed. Champaign, IL: Human Kinetics.

Hyatt, G. 1996. Strength training for the aging adult. *Activities, Adaptation & Aging* 20(3): 27-36.

Jacoby, S. 1999. Great sex: What's age got to do with it? The AARP/Modern Maturity survey on sexual attitudes and behavior. *Modern Maturity* (41)5: 91.

Jette, A.M., and L.G. Branch. 1981. The Framingham disability study: II—Physical disability among the aging. *American Journal of Public Health* 71: 11211-1216.

Joffe, H., A.N. Soares, and L.S. Cohen. 2003. Assessment and treatment of hot flashes and menopausal mood disturbance. *Psychiatric Clinics of North America* 26: 563-580.

Kemmler, W., K. Engleke, D. Lauber, J. Weineck, J. Hensen, and W.A. Kalener. 2002. Exercise effects on fitness and bone mineral density in early postmenopausal women: 1-year EFOPS results. *Medicine & Science in Sports & Exercise* 34(12): 2115-2123.

Kemmler, W., D. Lauber, J. Weineck, J. Hensen, W. Kalender, and K. Engleke. 2004. Benefits of 2 years of intense exercise on bone density, physical fitness, and blood lipids in early postmenopausal osteopenic women. *Archives of Internal Medicine* 164: 1084-1091.

Kerr, D., T. Ackland, B. Maslen, A. Morton, and R. Prince. 2001. Resistance training over 2 years increases bone mass in calcium-replete postmenopausal women. *Journal of Bone and Mineral Research* 16(1): 175-181.

Knudson, D. 1999. Stretching during warm-up: Do we have enough evidence? *Journal of Physical Education, Recreation & Dance* 70: 271-277.

Li, C.I., K.E. Malone, P.L. Porter, N.S. Weiss, M.C. Tang, K.L. Cushing-Haugen, and J.R. Daling. 2003. Relationship between long duration and different regimens of hormone therapy and risk of breast cancer. *Journal of the American Medical Association* 289(24): 3254-3263.

Littrell, T.R., and C.M. Snow. 2004. Bone density and physical function in postmenopausal women after a 12-month water exercise intervention. *Medicine & Science in Sports & Exercise* 36(5): S289 [Abstract].

Maglischo, E.W., and C.F. Brennan. 1985. *Swim for the health of it.* Palo Alto, CA: Mayfield.

Manson, J.E., P. Greenland, A.Z. LaCroix, M.L. Stefanick, C.P. Mouton, A. Oberman, M.G. Perri, D.S. Sheps, M.B. Pettinger, and D.S. Siscovick. 2002. Walking compared with vigorous exercise for the prevention of cardiovascular events in women. *New England Journal of Medicine* 347(10): 716-725.

Manson, J.E., J. Hsia, K.C. Johnson, J.E. Rossouw, A.R. Assaf, N.L. Lasser, J. Trevisan, H.R. Black, S.R. Heckbert, R. Detrano, O.L. Strickland, N.D. Wong, J.R. Crouse, E. Stein, and M. Cushman. 2003. Estrogen and progestin and the risk of coronary heart disease. *New England Journal of Medicine* 349(6): 523-534.

Manson, J.E., F.B. Hu, J.W. Rich-Edwards, G.A. Colditz, M.J. Stampfer, W.C. Willett, F.E. Speizer, and C.H. Hennekens. 1999. A prospective study of walking as compared with vigorous exercise in prevention of coronary heart disease in women. *New England Journal of Medicine* 341(9): 650-658.

Marcus, R. 2001. Role of exercise in preventing and treating osteoporosis. *Rheumatic Disease Clinics of North America* 27(1): 131-141.

McArdle, W.D., F.I. Katch, and V.L. Katch. 2001. *Exercise physiology: Energy, nutrition, and human performance.* 5th ed. Baltimore: Lippincott Williams & Wilkins.

McClung, M.R. 2003. Prevention and treatment of osteoporosis. *Best Practice and Research Clinical Endocrinology and Metabolism* 17(1): 53-71.

McTiernan, A., C. Kooperberg, E. White, S. Wilcox, R. Coates, L.L. Adams-Campbell, N. Woods, and J. Ockene. 2003. Recreational physical activity and the risk of breast cancer in postmenopausal women: The Women's Health Initiative cohort study. *Journal of the American Medical Association* 290(10): 1311-1336.

Midlife sexuality and women: Getting better with age. 2004. [Online]. Available: www.mayoclinic.com/invoke.cfm?id=HO00110 [June 19, 2004].

National Cholesterol Education Program. 1993. Report of the expert panel on population strategies for blood cholesterol reduction. *Archives of Internal Medicine* 148: 36-69.

National Institute on Aging. 2001. Exercise: A guide from the National Institute on Aging. NIH Publication No. 01-4258. Washington, DC: National Institute on Aging.

National Institutes of Health (NIH). 2003. The seventh report of the Joint National Committee on Prevention, Detection, Evaluation, and Treatment of High Blood Pressure. NIH Publication No. 03-5233. Washington, DC: NIH. [Online]. Available: http://www.nhlbi.nih.gov/guidelines/hypertension/express.pdf [November 10, 2004].

———. 2002. Women's health and menopause: A comprehensive approach. NIH Publication No. 02-3284. Washington, DC: National Institutes of Health.

———. 2001a. Menopause. U.S. Department of Health and Human Services, NIH Publication No. 01-3886. Washington, DC: National Institutes of Health.

———. 2001b. The third report of the National Cholesterol Education Program Expert Panel on Detection, Evaluation, and Treatment of Blood Cholesterol in Adults. NIH Publication No. 01-3760. Washington, DC: NIH. [Online]. Available: http://www.nhlbi.nih.gov/guidelines/cholesterol/atp3xsum.pdf [November 10, 2004].

———. 1997. NCI promotes proven benefits of mammography. National Institutes of Health News & Features, NIH Publication No. 98-3516. Washington, DC: National Institutes of Health.

———. 1994. Optimal calcium intake. NIH consensus statement online; 12(4): 1-31. Bethesda, MD: National Institutes of Health.

National Osteoporosis Foundation. 2002. Osteoporosis disease statistics 2002. [Online]. Available: www.nof.org [June 19, 2004].

Nelson, M.E., M.A. Fiatarone, C.M. Morganti, I. Trice, R.A. Greenberg, and W.J. Evans. 1994. Effects of high-intensity strength training on multiple risk factors for osteoporotic fractures: A randomized controlled trial. *Journal of the American Medical Association* 272(24): 1909-1914.

Nelson, M.E., and R. Sequin. 2004. Targeted exercise for promoting bone health in women. *American Journal of Medicine & Sports* 6(2): 94-96.

Nieman, D.C. 1999. *Exercise testing and prescription: A health-related approach.* 4th ed. Mountain View, CA: Mayfield.

North American Menopause Society (NAMS). 2004. Treatment of menopause-associated vasomotor symptoms: Position stand of the North American Menopause Society. *Menopause* 11(1): 11-33.

———. 2003. *Menopause guidebook: Helping women make informed healthcare decisions through perimenopause and beyond.* Cleveland: North American Menopause Society.

Osteoporosis Prevention, Diagnosis, and Therapy: NIH Consensus Development Panel on Osteoporosis Prevention, Diagnosis, and Therapy. 2001. *Journal of the American Medical Association* 285(6): 785-795.

Purdie, D.W. 1999. Raloxifene: Safety considerations and side-effects. In *The menopause at the millennium,* ed. T. Aso, T. Yanaihara, and S. Fujimoto, 484-485. New York: Parthenon.

Ross, M. 1999. Delayed-onset muscle soreness. *Physician and Sportsmedicine.* 29(13). [Online]. Available: www.physsportsmed.com/issues/1999/01_99/muscle.htm [February 2, 2004].

Sanders, M.E. 2000. *YMCA water fitness for health.* Champaign, IL: Human Kinetics.

Shangold, M.M., and C. Sherman. 1998. Exercise for midlife women. *Physician and Sportsmedicine.* 26(12). [Online]. Available: www.physsportsmed.com/issues/1998/12dec/shang_pa.htm [February 2, 2004].

Singh, M.A. 2000. *Exercise, nutrition, and the older woman.* Boca Raton, FL: CRC Press.

Staessen, J.A., G. Ginocchio, L. Thijs, and R. Fagard. 1997. Conventional and ambulatory blood pressure and menopause in a prospective population study. *Journal of Human Hypertension* 11: 507.

Stampfer, M.J., F.B. Hu, J.E. Manson, E.B. Rimm, and W.C. Willett. 2000. Primary prevention of coronary heart disease in women through diet and lifestyle. *New England Journal of Medicine* 343(1): 16-22.

Stearns, V., K.L. Beebe, M. Iyengar, and E. Dube. 2003. Paroxetine controlled release in the treatment of menopausal hot flashes: A randomized controlled trial. *Journal of the American Medical Association* 289(21): 2827-2834.

Teoman, N., A. Ozcan, and B. Acar. 2004. The effect of exercise on physical fitness and quality of life in postmenopausal women. *Maturitas* 47: 71-77.

Thune, I., T. Brenn, E. Lund, and M. Gaard. 1997. Physical activity and the risk of breast cancer. *New England Journal of Medicine* 336(18): 1269-1275.

US Department of Health and Human Services (US DHHS). 1996. *Physical activity and health: A report of the surgeon general.* Atlanta: Centers for Disease Control and Prevention, National Center for Chronic Disease Prevention and Health Promotion.

Wardlaw, G.M. 2003. *Contemporary nutrition.* 5th ed. New York: McGraw-Hill.

Wassertheil-Smoller, S., S.L. Hendrix, M. Limacher, G. Heiss, C. Kooperberg, A. Baird, T. Kotchen, J.D. Curb, H. Black, J.E. Rossouw, A. Aragaki, M. Safford, E. Stein, S. Laowattana, and W.J. Mysiw. 2003. Effect of estrogen plus progestin on stroke in postmenopausal women: The Women's Health Initiative: A randomized trial. *Journal of the American Medical Association* 289(20): 2673-2684.

Westcott, W.L., and T.R. Baechle. 1998. *Strength training past 50.* Champaign, IL: Human Kinetics.

Williams, M.H. 2002. *Nutrition for health, fitness & sport.* 6th ed. Boston: McGraw-Hill.

Willoughby, D.S. 2001. Resistance training in the older adult. *Current Comments From the American College of Sports Medicine.* April. [Online]. Available: www.acsm.org/health+fitness/pdf/currentcomments/rtoa.pdf [June 19, 2004].

Wilson, M-M.G. 2003. Menopause. *Clinics in Geriatric Medicine* 19: 483-506.

Women's Health Initiative Steering Committee. 2004. Effects of conjugated equine estrogen in postmenopausal women with hysterectomy: The Women's Health Initiative randomized controlled trial. *Journal of the American Medical Association* 291(14): 1701-1712.

Writing Group for the Women's Health Initiative. 2002. Risks and benefits of estrogen plus progestin in healthy postmenopausal women: Principal results from the Women's Health Initiative randomized controlled trial. *Journal of the American Medical Association* 288(3): 321-333.

INDEX

Note: The italicized *f* and *t* following page numbers refer to figures and tables, respectively.

ABOUT THE AUTHORS

Barbara Bushman is certified as a program director and exercise specialist through the American College of Sports Medicine (ACSM) and is an associate professor at Southwest Missouri State University. She received her PhD in exercise physiology from the University of Toledo and has since focused her research efforts on the topic of women and exercise, along with the usefulness of various exercise modes including cross-training and deep-water run training. Her findings have been featured in numerous journals, publications, and presentations.

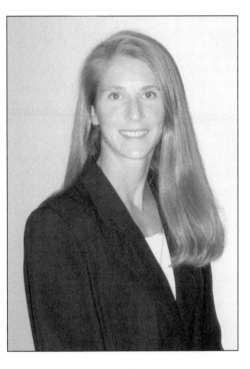

Bushman also is a manuscript reviewer for ACSM's *Medicine & Science in Sports & Exercise*, and she was a member of the editorial board of *The American Journal of Medicine & Sports*. She has been a fellow of the American College of Sports Medicine since 1999, serving on the ACSM Media Referral Network and ACSM's Strategic Health Initiative on Women, Sport and Physical Activity, along with various other national and regional ACSM committees.

Bushman resides in Springfield, Missouri, with her husband, Tobin, and participates in numerous activities in her leisure time, including running, cycling, hiking, lifting weights, and open-water kayaking.

Janice Clark Young is an assistant professor in the health and exercise sciences program at Truman State University in Kirksville, Missouri, where she teaches environmental health, program planning and evaluation, and consumer health. She earned her doctorate in health education from the University of Kansas and is a nationally certified health education specialist (CHES).

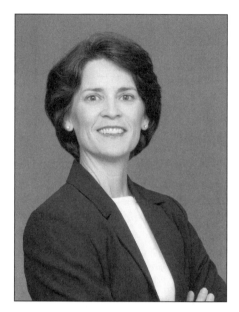

In addition to serving as a reviewer for six different health textbooks, Young also wrote the *Instructor's Manual for Hales' Invitation to Fitness and Wellness*. She is a member of the American Alliance for Health, Physical Education, Recreation and Dance and the American Association for Health Education. In 2003 she was the recipient of the College Teaching Award at Southwest Missouri State University.

Young resides in Kirksville, Missouri, with her husband, Frank. She enjoys a range of physical activities including swimming and water sports, horseback riding, dancing, and walking.

ABOUT THE ACSM

The **American College of Sports Medicine (ACSM)** is an association of more than 20,000 international, national, and regional chapter members in 80 countries. It is internationally known as the leading source of state-of-the-art research and information on sports medicine and exercise science. Learn about health and fitness, nutrition, sport-specific training and injuries, and more on the ACSM Web site: www.acsm.org.

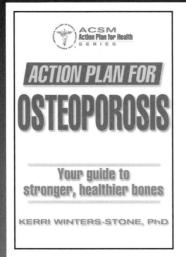
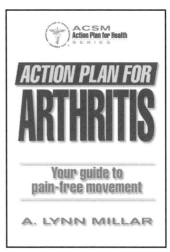